Abortion and the
Private Practice
of Medicine

Abortion and the Private Practice of Medicine

Jonathan B. Imber

Yale University Press
New Haven and London

Designed by Nancy Ovedovitz and set in
Galliard type by David E. Seham Associates,
Inc. Printed in the United States of America by
Vail-Ballou Press, Binghamton, N.Y.

**Library of Congress Cataloging-in-
Publication Data**

Imber, Jonathan B., 1952–
    Abortion and the private practice of medicine.
    Bibliography: p.
    Includes index.
    1. Abortion—United States.
2. Obstetrics—Decision making.
3. Abortion—Moral and ethical aspects.
4. Obstetricians—United States—Interviews.
5. Gynecologists—United States—Interviews.
I. Title. [DNLM: 1. Abortion, Induced—
United States.   2. Ethics, Medical—United
States.   3. Family Planning—United States.
4. Private Practice—United States.
HQ 767.5.U5 I32a]
RG734.I48   1986   179'.76   85-26528
ISBN 0-300-03554-3 (alk. paper)

RG
734
.I48
1986

The paper in this book meets the guidelines for
permanence and durability of the Committee on
Production Guidelines for Book Longevity of
the Council on Library Resources.

10   9   8   7   6   5   4   3   2   1

To my mother and father

The obstetrician . . . is concerned with the physical and mental welfare, the woes, the emotions, and the concern of his female patients. He, perhaps more than anyone else, is knowledgeable in this area of patient care, and he is aware of human frailty, so-called "error," and needs. The good physician—despite the presence of rascals in the medical profession, as in all others, we trust that most physicians are "good"—will have a sympathy and an understanding for the pregnant patient that probably is not exceeded by those who participate in other areas of professional counseling.

United States Supreme Court,
Doe v. Bolton [January 22, 1973]

Well, as it pleases them; I have not thrust my services on them; if they misuse me for sacred ends, I let that happen to me too.

Kafka, "A Country Doctor"

In a case like this I know
quick action is the main thing.

William Carlos Williams, "A Cold Front"

Contents

Preface

Abortion is the most frequently performed surgery in the United States today. Obstetrician/gynecologists (ob/gyns) are primarily responsible for performing the procedure, yet most ob/gyns perform only a small number of abortions—if any—in each year. In what follows, I explore the nature of obstetrical conservatism and its relation to the provision of abortion and family-planning services. Between 1978 and 1982, I conducted interviews with twenty-six ob/gyns who practiced in an eastern city I call Daleton. Their comments about their medical work and responsibilities form the major part of this book.[1]

Chapters 1 and 2 attempt to clarify abortion as a medical responsibility. At the beginning of the twentieth century, the law in effect did not permit abortion except to save a mother's life. Physicians were held responsible for determining when the procedure was warranted. After World War II, medical responsibility for abortion was formalized by the introduction of "therapeutic abortion committees" within the administration of hospitals. *Doe v. Bolton*, one of the two major decisions about abortion handed down by the Supreme Court in 1973, successfully challenged this system of decision making. The Court, in striking down all state laws prohibiting abortion, stipulated in *Doe v. Bolton* that the individual physician should be free to determine whether to perform the operation. The companion case, *Roe v. Wade*, affirmed a woman's "right to privacy."

Freed from the constraints of law and committees, some individuals began an organized effort to provide abortion services throughout the United States. Some residency programs, especially in the larger urban areas, became prototypes for what I call the culture of clinics, an environment in which virtually no request for abortion is denied. Such environments were also created by the establishment of free-standing abortion clinics. By 1976, 18 percent of all abortion providers performed 61 percent of all abortions (Sullivan *et al.*, 1977; see also Forrest *et al.*, 1978). The *New York Times* in March 1978 reported that of the million and more legal abortions performed in 1977, nearly 75 percent were performed in 250 of the estimated 500 clinics across the country (Wattleton and Kissling, 1978; see also Forrest *et al.*, 1979b).

This book does not address the culture of clinics, except to contrast in theoretical terms an institutional arrangement that affords the greatest possible access to abortion with the private practice of medicine, which does not. Outside the culture of clinics, ob/gyns practicing alone or in groups perform the remaining abortions either in hospitals or in their offices. Daleton had and continues to have no abortion clinic, although clinics can be found within thirty miles. The absence of a local clinic is an important aspect of the practice of obstetrics and gynecology in Daleton.

Chapters 3 to 6 report on the structure of private practice in obstetrics and gynecology in Daleton. I describe how the twenty-five men and one woman in that specialty, who ranged in age from thirty-one to sixty-seven and who were Protestants, Catholics, and Jews, viewed their personal and professional responsibilities toward family planning, abortion, and the practice of medicine. The opportunity to meet and learn more about these doctors was unique. My being a male was no doubt helpful when asking questions of men about a matter that impinges so differently on women. My prior familiarity with the community gave me access to physicians who might otherwise have been "too busy" to talk to a researcher. Many doctors conversed with me at length about the community and about their medical practices; others would not elaborate on their answers. The reticence of some and the enthusiastic participation of others reflected, in part, who each was in his or her practice of medicine. Often they expressed to me beliefs and feelings that were generally known to their colleagues but were rarely shared explicitly.

This book has more to say about doctors' responsibilities toward the practice of medicine than about the politics, law, or ethics of abortion. It began with the opposite focus, only to come face to face with the issue of practice. As a graduate student in sociology, I studied the emerging field known as bioethics, which has since given rise to academic and public institutes, government commissions, annual meetings and retreats, and an orchestrated attempt to bring ethics to medicine. I remember attending a lecture by one of the better-known figures in bioethics given at Daleton's largest hospital. His intention was to offer physicians, nurses, and hospital administrators a framework for assessing ethical dilemmas in the delivery of health care. Not one of the ob/gyns attended; in fact, the audience appeared to include more people out of white than in white.

At the time, in the very early stages of my interviewing, I began to realize that my questions to physicians were not as relevant to them as I had thought they would be, given the intense public and intellectual scrutiny of abortion. Asking a doctor to recite the basic principles of *Roe v. Wade* and *Doe v. Bolton* proved to be not only off the point but also an impoverished way of talking about medicine. Fortunately, as often happens in the course of fieldwork, in my questions I soon began to follow the respondents' answers more than the interview schedule. The practice of medicine was not a series of intellectual debates about ethics and law but a way of acting with patients, colleagues, and, importantly, family.

Some of the constraints on the work of physicians in private practice were self-imposed; others were consequences of developments in research medicine and epidemiology. In chapters 5 and 6, I argue that epidemiological knowledge about the safety and effectiveness of different procedures and medicines, including methods for second-trimester abortion and the contraceptive pill, play a crucial, but sometimes ambiguous, role in physicians' medical practices. What was resolved at the aggregate level as scientific fact was not neatly translated to the experiences and understandings of doctors in their everyday practices. As persons, these physicians were caught in a web of circumstances that this study seeks to make more explicit.

The private practice of medicine continues to offer doctors a shield against public scrutiny of their actions. As a refuge from controversial innovations within the practice of medicine and from political forces outside the profession, private practice in Daleton was the central institutional means that enabled physicians to determine what kinds of services they would and would not offer.

Why talk with physicians about abortion? As a political issue, legal access to abortion is of paramount concern to many, whether they favor or oppose it. By focusing on physicians, I do not mean to diminish the importance of women's reactions to and experiences with abortion. But a woman's right to choose the procedure is always circumscribed by the physician's right not to perform it. The social organization of abortion services in the United States has been criticized by some who believe that physicians should be more responsive to the interests of women as patients. Diana Scully, for instance, has concluded: "Self-determination for women is not likely to become a major goal of the specialty soon." She questions the "monopoly" on abortion exercised by ob/gyns without considering that its performance may be problematic for any group, even ones "psychologically better prepared for the work" (1980:90). The preparation required has not been easily accomplished even within the culture of clinics.[2]

My own feelings are important to express. An issue that so deeply divides people cannot be worked through by ignoring the force of those feelings in oneself or others. If a referendum were taken tomorrow proposing to make abortion illegal again, I would vote against it. I believe the consequences would be far worse than many in the pro-life movement are willing to admit. Nevertheless, the heart of the matter is that our society stands witness to well over one million abortions each year. For many patients and doctors, abortion is a personal tragedy and an individually agonizing decision to make. From a societal standpoint, however, its routine accomplishment is now an accepted fact of life.

The deliberate resort to abortion is a failing, not an inevitable consequence, of how we live. Until very recently, this moral valuation was unchallenged. Even Havelock Ellis, who today would be canonized as a saint of sexual liberation, remarked on abortion at the beginning of this century:

> The progress of civilization is in the direction of greater foresight, of greater prevention, of a diminished need for struggling with the reckless lack of prevision. The necessity of abortion is precisely one of those results of reckless action which civilization tends to diminish. While we may admit that in a sounder state of civilization a few cases might still occur when the induction of abortion would be desirable, it seems probable that the number of such cases will decrease rather than increase. (1913:611)

Ellis spoke during a time when opponents of birth control intentionally confused it with abortion. Today the struggle over the control of birth has shifted from moral valuations of specific forms of birth control to social movements asserting the inalienable rights of individuals, living and unborn.

The debate over abortion, sociologist Kristin Luker (1984b) has recently argued, is symbolic of a split between two world views about sex roles, parenthood, and human nature. For an understanding of social trends, these world views are more relevant to the sociologist than the philosophical and legal conundrums of abortion. Yet more than world views are at stake in the continuing debate about this ancient form of birth control.

The modern accomplishment of a premeditated control of events in life transcends the world views of those who disagree about the best ways to meet the responsibilities of parenthood. Such control on a mass scale would be unimaginable without the participation of a specially trained elite. For a time, abortion connoted a loss of the rational control of reproduction. As this connotation recedes in the light of claims that abortion is a relatively safe and efficient form of birth control, the medical profession becomes increasingly instrumental for its provision. The vast use of abortion today demonstrates the failure of public efforts to educate people toward a higher responsibility in the control of conception. Those who are resigned to this failure accept statistical fact as a mandate on human nature: the prospect for a reduction in the numbers of abortions will remain dim indeed as long as it is assumed that human beings cannot do better for themselves.

This book is addressed to many constituencies in the abortion debate: to those in the pro-life and pro-choice movements, to religious fundamentalists, to feminists and radical feminists, to bioethicists, and to those caught between the politics and practicalities of social welfare. Beyond the politics of abortion, the doctor's dilemma has persisted for centuries. Medical practice remains a moral domain insofar as physicians' responsibilities have been neither completely dictated nor fully determined. The distinctively modern hope to reconcile innovation in technique with human fallibility may eventually result in further control of physicians by forces beyond medicine. In the meantime, the practice of medicine has proved to be remarkably resilient, despite the continuing pressures on physicians to conform to the politics of one side or the other.

Acknowledgments

I began this book as a doctoral dissertation under the supervision of Philip Rieff, Renée C. Fox, and E. Digby Baltzell of the University of Pennsylvania. Philip Rieff taught me the inescapable pressure of the theoretical life; he patiently repeated (and still does) the importance of seeing theory as a vision of the highest and not merely as a system of ideas. A follow-up study was then supported by the James Picker Foundation Program for the Human Qualities of Medicine under the direction of Renée C. Fox. I am grateful to Renée Fox for her confidence and friendship over the past ten years. Her invitation to me to join the Picker Foundation Program offered an opportunity for important discussions about the practice of medicine. This book owes much to those discussions, and I would like to thank Jean and Harvey Picker for helping to make it possible. Charles Bosk, Willy De Craemer, and Henry Erle took a special interest in my work during that time.

I am indebted to many others for their encouragement and criticism, and in particular to Brigitte Berger, Samuel W. Bloom, Lee Cuba, H. Tristram Engelhardt, Douglas A. Harper, Rosanna Hertz, Leon R. Kass, Barbara Kaye, Howard Kaye, Parker G. Marden, Len M. Nichols, and Eviatar Zerubavel. Without the help of Georgie M. Duquet and Richard C. Schofield, the computer-assisted production of manuscript would not have run so smoothly.

My first teacher in sociology, Kurt H. Wolff, has remained for fifteen years a constant guide and source of inspiration. I am thankful for his and Carla E. Wolff's support, questions, and understanding.

I wish to thank Alan N. Woolfolk for his untiring efforts in helping me make sense of it all and John T. Fidler, whose long friendship has made the effort worthwhile. Gladys Topkis offered superb assistance in her editing and questioning, and I am grateful to her and to Alexander Metro of Yale University Press.

The doctors of Daleton, who all remain anonymous in what follows, gave generously of themselves, and they were gracious when I reappeared, in some cases several times, to ask more about their work. I trust that what I say about them and about their community will contribute to a better understanding of the doctor's vocation.

Finally, I am blessed with parents who have supported me in all ways possible. So has my wife, Amy, who inspires me to write further about the meaning of vocation; half that meaning would be lost without her.

1
Abortion as a Medical Responsibility

Until recently, abortion was one of the most widely proscribed practices in Western culture. The Hippocratic oath specifically prohibited it, and this injunction was supported by Judeo-Christian reverence for life. With the legalization of abortion in many parts of the world during the twentieth century, this barrier has given way to such an extent that the physician's responsibility for deciding whether to perform the procedure is now seen to be of less consequence for its availability than the outcome of political struggles that may have little to do with medicine.

Birth *control,* as it was called by such leaders of contemporary Western sexual enlightenment as Margaret Sanger, offered a new sovereignty over unborn life, first to women and then to the medical profession and the state. For half a century the birth control movement publicly maintained the moral distinction between contraception and abortion, extolling the former while condemning the latter as barbaric and unnecessary. The rhetoric called for a pedagogy that would instruct patients (that is, women) and doctors in the responsible control of conception (see Kennedy, 1970; Gordon, 1976; and Reed, 1978). Until the early 1970s, the rubric *family planning* concealed a change in attitudes that had taken place among supporters of birth control who also endorsed a less inhibited sexuality. With the rise of the contemporary women's movement, the right to obtain an abortion became a prerequisite to the liberation of women. The assertion that control over one's body must include the right to choose abortion was quickly countered by the assertion that the taking of life is never permissible.

Discussion of abortion extends far back in the history of Western religious thought, and for many the matter continues to be a troubling spiritual problem (Noonan, 1970; Jakobovits, 1975; Connery, 1977). Ignorance about the biological origins and development of life also resulted in many differences of opinion about the circumstances in which abortion should be permitted. But with the rise of scientific medicine in the nineteenth century, a new consensus began to form among physicians.

In the United States, abortion was not punishable by statute before 1820, although the common law had provided penalties for the destruction of unborn life after the time of "quickening," or that moment in pregnancy when the mother first experiences the movement of the fetus. By 1890 every state in the nation had passed a law prohibiting abortion. Historian James C. Mohr has demonstrated persuasively that in the mid-nineteenth century the "graduates of the country's better medical schools" and the members of the newly established (1847) American Medical Association led the campaign to outlaw abortion in America (1978:33–34; 147–48). These so-called regular doctors assumed an authority over the procedure that has had a lasting effect on the moral connotations of the term *abortionist,* despite dramatic changes in the law in recent years.

Mohr's study presents important revisions in our understanding of traditional resistances to the practice of abortion. The "regulars" moved against it, he argues, in order to use state power to enhance their control over the practice of medicine by those who lacked their credentials. The claim that the medical profession had the central role in this effort is supported by the apparent lack of public, and especially Protestant, opposition to abortion. Although the Catholic Church has consistently opposed abortion, for Mohr the pro-choice view that gained prominence in the 1970s can be interpreted as a continuation of the public indifference of the nineteenth century and as further evidence that abortion is neither abhorrent nor spiritually troublesome to large segments of the population. This revisionist view has found confirmation in recent changes in the law.

Mohr describes the medical profession's allegiance to the newly emerging ideology of the scientific treatment of disease. Scientific research, technical expertise, and standardized treatment were expected to reduce the fallibility of human judgment. The opposition to abortion was thus led by a professional guild that sought legal and cultural hegemony over medical procedures, but did so in the name of science.[1]

Nineteenth-century American doctors' efforts to restrict abortion were indebted to a growing understanding of fetal development, as yet unknown to the lay population: "Scientifically, regulars had realized for some time that conception inaugurated a more or less continuous process of development which would produce a new human being if uninterrupted. . . . From this scientific reasoning stemmed the regulars' moral opposition to abortion at any stage in gestation" (Mohr, 1978:35–36). Further: "Most physicians considered abortion a crime because of the inherent difficulties of determining any point at which a steadily developing embryo became somehow more alive than it had been the moment before" (1978:165). The cultural resistance to abortion in America originated not in public opinion or in particular theological doctrine as much as in the medical profession's commitment to scientific findings. Against the amoral image of science that Max Weber (1948) bequeathed to modernity, nineteenth-century science produced extraordinary moments of clarity in the relation between facts and values. Instead of creating new exceptions to the laws prohibiting abortion, the scientific knowledge of conception formed the basis for a powerful opposition to it and strengthened theological valuations of the sanctity of unborn life. Faced with the knowledge that a human life is developing from the moment of conception, regular doctors publicly opposed the resort to abortion. A major purpose of this chapter is to review how physicians went about determining exceptions to the rule that prohibited them from interrupting pregnancy.

The work of Dr. Frederick Joseph Taussig (1872–1943) during the first half of the twentieth century exemplifies the way in which many physicians construed their responsibilities regarding the performance of abortion. Educated at Harvard and at the Washington University Medical School, Taussig taught and practiced obstetrics and gynecology for most of his life in St. Louis. He was president of the American Gynecological Society (1936–37) and director of the American Society for the Control of Cancer (1938). His prominence in American obstetrics and gynecology was firmly established by the publication of several books, especially *Diseases of the Vulva* (1923) and *Abortion, Spontaneous and Induced: Medical and Social Aspects* (1936). (See Crossen, 1943, and Marquis, 1943, 1945).

In *Criminal Abortion: A Study in Medical Sociology* (1964), Jerome E. Bates and Edward S. Zawadzki wrote:

> It is a relatively recent event to have physicians of national reputation speaking and writing on the social repercussions of our abortion laws. Frederick J. Taussig, M.D., pioneered in this field by publishing *Abortion: Spontaneous and Induced* in 1936. This work was primarily a medical book with a few chapters covering induced abortion from a sociological and historical point of view. As one might expect the book had no effect on the public although it did encourage other physicians to study the effects of criminal abortion on maternal and child welfare. (p. 115)

Bates and Zawadzki did not mention (except in their bibliography) that Taussig had written *The Prevention and Treatment of Abortion* many years earlier, in 1910. This work was the first full-length study in twentieth-century America of the "anatomy, pathology, etiology, and diagnosis of this condition" (p. 2).

The book addressed three important aspects of the abortion problem. First, Taussig's analysis of the medical indications that justified therapeutic abortion guided discussions by later American physicians. Second, his remarks about the prevention of conception anticipated the role that contraception would eventually play in American medicine. And third, his thoughts on the prevention of criminal abortion offered valuable insights into the dilemma of how best to reduce the use of abortion as a means of birth control.

A distinction between therapeutic and nontherapeutic abortion has always existed in medical parlance. Both types are called induced abortions in that birth would result if pregnancy were otherwise undisturbed. According to Taussig, "Therapeutic abortion has been defined as the induction of abortion on the part of the physician in order to save the life of the mother" (1910:162). He listed three general categories of medical indications for the procedure:

1. pathologic conditions due directly to the pregnancy,
2. maternal diseases aggravated by pregnancy, and
3. extreme contractions of the birth canal.

Of the three pathologic conditions that he cited, "incarceration of the pregnant uterus," he said, "is most often due to retroflexion or retroversion of the gravid uterus" (1910:162). In other words, the pregnant uterus is bent in such a way that it cannot assume its proper shape, thus imperiling the lives of the mother and of the unborn child. He proposed several ways to alleviate the condition, the most radical of which was hysterectomy, or removal of the entire uterus. Laparotomy, which required incision through the abdominal flank in order to reach and "break up the dense adhesions that bound down the uterus," was also recommended before resort to a therapeutic abortion (1910:163).

Acute hydramnios, or excessive buildup of amniotic fluid in the uterus, could not only cause severe pain but result in cardiac insufficiency, making therapeutic abortion "absolutely necessary" and the likelihood of a live birth "practically nil" (1910:163). The third pathologic condition, "one of the most frequent and important indications for therapeutic abortions," was hyperemesis, or excessive vomiting. This was occasionally misleading, Taussig noted, because "vomiting is at times brought on by the patient so as to influence the physician to hasten the emptying of the uterus." He advised that such a patient be placed in a hospital and "kept under constant watch." Referring to a report in the medical literature, he described a patient "who by persistent vomiting and by abstaining from food lost thirty-seven pounds in four weeks. After the doctor had finally felt compelled to do an abortion, she laughingly remarked to him that she could have refrained from vomiting if she cared to" (1910:163). Taussig warned that "one has to be on guard against such malingerers" (1910:164).

The second group of indications for therapeutic abortion consisted of those maternal diseases that were sometimes aggravated by pregnancy, "primarily *heart* and *kidney* lesions and *tuberculosis* of the respiratory tract" (1910:164). In these cases, therapeutic abortion did not treat the ailment but reduced the likelihood that it would become life-threatening. Taussig also believed that "certain nervous and psychic diseases at times necessitate the induction of abortion. Not, however, the neurasthenias or even the cases of so-called nervous prostration" (1910:164–65). The fatigue and mental depression often associated with pregnancy, he concluded, were not sufficient indications of the need for therapeutic abortion.

The final group of indications, "marked narrowing of the birth canal," referred to "cases where Caesarian section is absolutely necessary for the delivery of a living child" (1910:165). Taussig recommended that the mother be permitted to decide whether she would undergo a Caesarian section, but he added: "As a rule, if she is in fair general condition she should be persuaded to await the end of pregnancy and have a Caesarian section performed, since statistics show that this operation is attended with a very small mortality" (1910:165). In a case he described as "inoperable cancer of the cervix," Taussig saw no justification for terminating the pregnancy, "since here the mother's life is lost anyway and every effort must be made to get a living child by Caesarian section" (ibid.). It is worth noting that Taussig viewed Caesarian section as a way of avoiding the resort to induced abortion earlier in the pregnancy. Hysterotomy or a "mini-Caesarian" section, sometimes used as a method for late second-trimester abortion, was not yet discussed, in large part because the physician's obligation was to encourage the continuation of pregnancy until a living child could be delivered.

The medical indications that Taussig described may be said to have *compelled* the physician to perform an abortion, but only after other avenues of care had proved ineffective. Therapeutic abortion was most strongly indicated during medical emergency when the mother's life was clearly in jeopardy. Although maternal diseases of the heart, lungs, and kidneys were sometimes aggravated by pregnancy, they represented weaker indications for abortion than more immediately life-threatening disorders. For Taussig, the physician's medical judgment embodied his particular understanding of disease and its potential effect on both the mother's health and her pregnancy. How "medical" indications were to be defined became more difficult to determine in cases of "certain nervous and psychic diseases" and "so-called nervous prostration."

At the beginning of the twentieth century, the practice of abortion was regarded by the general public as a criminal activity regardless of the medical indications for the interruption of pregnancy. For at least the next sixty years, the social fact of abortion's illegality—what Taussig described as "the odium attaching to the name" (1910:2)—would remain its most conspicuous feature. Indeed, as has been noted, one of the strategies of the leaders of the birth control movement was to distinguish their call for the dissemination of birth control information from any support for the legalization of abortion (Imber, 1979:825). Abortion was universally regarded as the most drastic and most dangerous form of birth control, and the advocates of birth control hoped that improved contraceptive knowledge would help to prevent it. Taussig anticipated the general acceptance by most physicians of the preventive uses of contraception, and he chided his colleagues for not taking greater responsibility for such education:

> There is a natural reluctance on the part of physicians and text-books to discuss this subject, since it is apt to lead to abuses in one way or another. And yet, this very refusal on the part of the profession to speak of these subjects has led to the most serious mistakes and injurious practices on the part of their patients. There has been much prudery and prejudice in the views of Americans on this subject. (1910:167)

Of "the most frequently practiced" forms of contraception, Taussig claimed that coitus interruptus "leads in time to chronic congestion of the organs of reproduction and to certain nervous disturbances, often of a serious character" (1910:168). He criticized the "stem pessary" (a precursor of the modern intrauterine device), insisting that it was "in fact, rather an abortifacient than a means of avoiding conception" (ibid.).

Taussig's remarks in 1910 may have struck many of his fellow doctors as unorthodox, but they were clearly derived from his clinical experience. Most of the criminal abortions he and his colleagues were compelled to complete, he believed, could have been prevented. It would always be an essential part of the training of obstetrician/gynecologists (ob/gyns) to know how to treat an incomplete abortion, whether spontaneous or induced. But in the case of botched abortion, this knowledge was helpful only after the fact. Taussig recognized that improved medical treatment of abortion had the unintended consequence of making the procedure a safer and therefore more reasonable form of birth control:

> The discovery of asepsis and antisepsis has not proved any unmixed blessing. Criminal abortion can at the present time be done with less danger of blood-poisoning than formerly. The result is inevitable. One of the main deterrent factors in the production of abortion is gone when the woman realizes that her own life is not necessarily imperiled. (1910:78–79)

A new public perception of risk slowly emerged from the once discouraging fear of being injured or dying from an illegally induced
abortion. Taussig knew that physicians would be ethically compelled
to treat the sequelae of badly performed abortions. He also understood that criminal abortion was bound to increase because of the
improvement in the performance of abortions and the treatment of
poorly performed ones.

Taussig concluded: "It seems probable that this question [criminal
abortion] will become one of the most serious sociological problems
of the coming years, for every community must in self-preservation
enact laws and exert its utmost influence to stem this tide that will
otherwise sweep it to destruction" (1910:79). He proposed that new
educational strategies be developed to discourage women from seeking abortions:

> The myth that life does not begin until fetal movements are felt is still so
> widespread that it will take many years before it is finally put aside. Almost
> daily the physician hears the story that the woman did not think it was
> wrong to stop pregnancy in the early months before the child was alive. . . .
> Women of all classes should know more concerning the processes of ges-
> tation. They should be shown how early the fetal heart begins to pump
> blood through its vessels. (1910:79)

Taussig believed that the dissemination of medical-scientific knowledge about conception and fetal development might instill a new
fear in women who had believed that abortion was morally wrong
only after experiencing the sensation of fetal movement. This new
fear, he hoped, would counteract the effects of improvements in the
management of badly performed abortions, which might otherwise
lead to an increase in the resort to abortion.

Taussig's pedagogy of prevention relied not only on scientific facts
but also on effective presentation of the facts. He arranged a series
of medical lectures to be given by a nurse in one of the social set-
tlements of St. Louis. The nurse was instructed to use an enlarged
picture of an embryo of six weeks in order to emphasize "the fact
that at this time the eyes, ears, nose, mouth and extremities were
already crudely formed." Taussig stressed that "it is not enough merely
to tell them [women] that in producing an abortion in the early
months they are taking a human life; they must be shown that at
this period the child is already well along in its development. I think

pictures like that of the six weeks' embryo will keep many women from having an abortion done" (1910:79). The visual image of the embryo/fetus has remained to this day a potent symbol for those persuaded against abortion. The refinement of photographic technique now allows a view of the course of fetal development and of the burns and disarticulations of the fetal body caused by certain methods of termination (compare Nilsson, 1977, and Hilgers and Horan, 1972:297–99).[2]

For Taussig, the image of the developing fetus symbolized a new knowledge about aspects of human life that were a mystery for many in 1910. A half-century later, the wonder of creation would be carefully separated from the reality of creation aborted. As will be seen, the split in fetal images has institutional and professional analogues. The abortion clinic in American society sets itself apart from obstetric delivery and care, and obstetrician/gynecologists have found numerous ways to keep abortion practice isolated from obstetric practice.

In addition to advocating improved scientific education in order to reduce criminal abortion, Taussig called for legislative changes. He was convinced that if all abortions were officially reported, no matter what the cause, there would eventually be a reduction in the number of criminal abortions: "Moreover, independent of its effect upon this question, the government is entitled to know of the death of any living being, whether that being has advanced to full-term development or not. It is time that the antiquated ideas of modern law as to when life begins be modified in accordance with our present knowledge. Life begins with conception" (1910:81).

Taussig's recommendations intended an incorporation of scientific fact in legislative mandate. Yet, as the compilation of abortion statistics became a routine part of epidemiological record keeping, a new ideological justification for abortion was constructed: legally performed abortions were statistically safer than illegally performed ones. Taussig would not live to see his suggestion that all abortions be reported transformed into the epidemiological conclusion that the only way to reduce the number of criminal abortions was to allow the procedure to be performed in an expanded range of legal circumstances. His other recommendation, that the law incorporate the "present knowledge" that "life begins with conception," is now associated exclusively with the anti-abortion movement.

Both educational and legislative efforts to discourage the practice of abortion were undermined by innovations in medical technology. Taussig was willing to consider other ways of stemming the tide of abortion practice. Like many Americans during the 1920s and 1930s, he visited the Soviet Union in order to appraise the work of the Revolution. He was specifically interested in the effects of legal abortion on maternal health. His observations can be found in the pages of the *American Journal of Obstetrics and Gynecology* (1931a, 1931b, 1937). The Soviets legalized abortion in 1920, outlawed it again in 1936, and re-legalized it in 1955 (Field, 1956). Dissatisfaction with the Soviet government's response to the problem made Taussig more receptive to the strategy taken by leaders of the birth control movement, who heralded contraception as the only way to reduce the practice of abortion substantially (Taussig, 1936:405–420, and Imber, 1985).

At the American Medical Association meetings in June 1934, Taussig participated in a discussion about the medical indications for therapeutic abortion:

> To say that if the indications are hard and fast it leaves the door open to all kinds of abuses may to some extent be true, but all know that these abuses exist. Unscrupulous physicians readily find excuses for an abortion that is really done for other reasons. That is no reason for taking away from the conscientious physician the privilege of deciding each case on its own merits with that broader wisdom which seeks to act for the good health, happiness and proper care of that particular family. The number of cases that must be aborted have taken a definite drop, while the number of cases that may be aborted have at the same time increased. (1934:1918)

The "broader wisdom" that Taussig sought for all practitioners had two sources. First, there was the duty of each physician to "act for the good health, happiness and proper care" of each family. Second, that duty was to be exercised within the limits of what the physician defined as medical necessity. The broader wisdom would broaden further as the medical necessity for abortion was reduced. Between the two world wars, before abortion became a social problem that contraceptive education could not entirely solve, Taussig encouraged practitioners to exercise their "privilege of deciding" as they saw fit.

With the publication of Taussig's *Abortion, Spontaneous and Induced* in 1936, the physician's privilege became a matter for wider discussion and debate. The legal status of therapeutic abortion at that time can be summed up in the following way: six states provided no legal exemptions for intentionally induced abortion; 38 states recognized "saving the life of the mother" as the only legal exemption for induction; three states and the District of Columbia recognized "preservation of health" as an additional indication; and only one state, Mississippi, permitted abortion when deemed necessary by a physician (pp. 426–434).

Well versed in the literal meanings of the law, Taussig also knew that its spirit had been entrusted to his profession. As in his 1910 work, he analyzed the indications for therapeutic abortion and continued to defend the medical necessity for the interruption of pregnancy as the foundation of any practical understanding of the physician's responsibility. He criticized proposals for other indications made by Abraham Rongy in a controversial book entitled *Abortion: Legal or Illegal?* (1933). "In the propaganda for broader indications for the induction of abortion there have been some who have taken what seems to me an extreme point of view. I cannot agree with Dr. Rongy for instance when he advocates abortion in every case of illegitimacy or advises it in cases of desertion or widowhood" (1936:448). Viewing himself as a moderate against the strong progressive and eugenic propaganda for broader indications, Taussig proposed instead that the state should "make provision for the maternal and physical welfare of the newborn babe by adoption or by financial support, rather than . . . legalize its destruction before birth" (ibid.). He now admitted more candidly the need to assess factors besides medical indications in determining whether an abortion should be performed. The physician was expected to establish a balance between medical and nonmedical factors.

Taussig supported public sex education but once again chided his colleagues for not taking greater responsibilities along this line: "In daily office routine, a physician frequently has opportunities of discussing these subjects with his patients. He is not worthy of his calling who does not take the necessary time to do his work of education" (1936:449). In 1936, the same year in which Taussig's magnum opus appeared, the law was changed to allow physicians to dispense birth control more freely (Reed, 1978:121). Contraception became a state-supported virtue and thus a major goal of the birth control movement was achieved.

Taussig's mammoth study speculated on the incidence of abortion in America and surveyed its economic, domestic, theological, and ethical aspects. Years after its publication, this work continued to be referred to as the first major contribution to the view of abortion as a social, rather than strictly medical, problem.

By the mid-1930s, the reports by individual practitioners of their clinical experiences with abortion had begun to give way to large-scale studies that analyzed hundreds of cases at a time. The modern epidemiology of abortion took shape in this approach. Most of the studies presented reviews of therapeutic abortions done in hospital settings, though the earliest ones are accounts of the medical treatment of botched criminal abortions (Watkins, 1933; R. E. Stewart, 1935; Bearle, 1942; Sangmeister, 1943). The new attempt to observe patterns and regularities in the practice of abortion also produced broader agreement about the improved prospects for maternal health in general. Physicians could no longer appeal to a specific set of guidelines about when abortion was indicated since they could now treat most maternal disorders without having to resort to the procedure. As medical indications declined, they turned to hospital committees for confirmation and protection.

One significant statistical correlation was consistently made in articles published in the *American Journal of Obstetrics and Gynecology* (AJOG) between 1933 and 1939. In a "Statistical Analysis of One Thousand Abortions," Jalmar H. Simons concluded that among patients "religion does not seem to be a deterrent to induction of abortion" (1939:846).[3] Endre K. Brunner and Louis Newton reached a similar conclusion in "Abortions in Relation to Viable Births in 10,609 Pregnancies" (1939:90). If religion had ever served as a deterrent to abortion, these studies cited its contemporary irrelevance and recommended the need for improved contraceptive education.

By 1940, medical indications for abortion were being widely discussed in the literature. In "Limitation of Human Reproduction: Therapeutic Abortion," H. Close Hesseltine, F. L. Adair, and M. W. Boynton reported that 134 pregnancies had been terminated before the twenty-eighth week at the Chicago Lying-in Hospital between 1931 and 1939. The leading indication had been pulmonary tuberculosis, followed by rheumatic heart disease, chronic nephritis, neurologic and psychiatric disorders (including psychosis, psychoneurosis, epilepsy, and multiple sclerosis), hypertension, hyperemesis, pre-eclampsia, and a variety of other conditions, including arthritis and diabetes (1940:552). In discussions following the article, some disagreements were sounded about the induction of abortion in cases of psychosis. More important, a consensus was beginning to form about the necessity of having at least two other doctors in addition to the one attending the patient involved in the decision to terminate a pregnancy. In his closing remarks, Dr. Hesseltine noted: "The therapeutic abortion committee . . . is a very good idea. It would give moral support and medico-legal protection to the institution and to the individuals responsible" (1940:561). In the years that followed, support for this idea increased.

Virginia Clay Hamilton offered a major reformulation of abortion as a social problem in a series of three articles for AJOG in 1940 and 1941:

> That induced abortion is primarily a sociologic and psychologic problem is self-evident. If conditions did not exist which make offspring undesirable, to the particular woman at the particular time, there would be no induced abortion. If every married woman felt her family budget sufficient to provide satisfactorily for unlimited children, if there were no social stigma associated with illegitimacy, the incidence of induced abortion would, no doubt, be reduced to a fraction of its present magnitude. (1940:919)

Hamilton's approach, like most others', still centered on how the resort to abortion could be reduced. She proposed four "ultimate steps in the prevention of abortion":

1. Preferential community service to families with children.
2. Maternity leave for employed women.
3. Social and economic aid to unmarried pregnant women and responsible agencies to care for and place illegitimate children.
4. Sex education at all levels correlated with instruction in child care and cultivation of an understanding of the values of parenthood. (1940:927)

Hamilton presented new insights in two subsequent articles, "The Clinical and Laboratory Differentiation of Spontaneous and Induced Abortion" and the "Medical Status and Psychologic Attitude of Patients Following Abortion." The first of these articles reviewed 502 cases of women admitted to Bellevue Hospital, New York, with complications following spontaneous and induced abortions. Although nearly 70 percent of them stated that the abortion had been spontaneous, Hamilton noted that "a clean curettage by a skilled abortionist is obviously no more liable to infection than a therapeutic abortion performed in our own operating room" (1941a:62). On the other hand, an incomplete spontaneous abortion could easily be mistaken for an incompetently induced one. She concluded: "The uterus recognizes no moral distinctions" (1941a:63). Record keeping of abortions in hospitals was complicated by the fact that a patient's account was often more important than any laboratory technique in determining what type of abortion had occurred.

For her third article, Hamilton interviewed 100 women who returned for postoperative care after their stay at Bellevue about their feelings toward their partners, coitus, and abortion (1941b:286–287). The more complex understanding of motivating factors in both spontaneous and induced abortion invited new types of investigation of the abortion problem by social scientists as well as medical specialists. In the years that followed, the variable of psychological harm associated with induced abortion was often included in proposals for and against its wider accessibility.

Thomas V. Moore of the Catholic University of America contributed an article to the September 1940 issue of AJOG entitled "Moral Aspects of Therapeutic Abortion." He had presented it earlier in the year to a symposium on abortion at Johns Hopkins Medical School. A Benedictine monk and physician, Moore was the author of *Principles of Ethics* (1935), a major attempt to forge a philosophy of conduct with regard to medicine and nursing. His reflections on the medical and moral justifications for abortion, in both his book and his article, anticipated many of the opinions that were more popularly expressed in the 1970s by those in the right-to-life movement. In particular, Moore was probably the first to draw the analogy between the right to life with respect to people under dictatorship and the right to life with respect to the unborn (1940:428).[4]

Moore also discussed craniotomy, used to interrupt an advanced pregnancy to save the mother's life. The operation was said to involve two stages, the first requiring perforation of the skull of the fetus and the second calling for the "complete destruction of the cerebral contents" (1940:423) so that the fetus could be more easily removed. The second stage had become generally accepted "by reason of the fact that physicians from time to time were horrified by the delivery of a living child, in spite of the fact that much of its cerebral tissue had been destroyed" (ibid.). He proposed that "with its plastic nervous system [the child] might survive the loss of a considerable amount of cerebral tissue and still be able to develop a normal mental life" (ibid.).

Whether or not one subscribed to the long tradition in Catholic teaching on abortion, those trained in that tradition were able to make explicit the moral and medical dilemmas that physicians faced several decades later. The question of which procedure to use in second-trimester abortions in the 1970s and 1980s, examined in more detail in chapter 5, is reminiscent of Moore's discussion of craniotomy in the 1940s.

Nearly two-thirds of the articles published in the *American Journal of Obstetrics and Gynecology* during the 1940s made reference to Frederick Taussig's *Abortion, Spontaneous and Induced.* By 1943, AJOG had added to its regular features a "Department of Statistics," another sign that the epidemiological approach was gradually replacing the narrower definition of abortion as a medical and moral problem for individual practitioners.

Yet concern about the practitioner's responsibility persisted in other forms in the professional literature, as is seen in a controversy over hospital policy regarding the performance of therapeutic abortion. In the September 1944 issue of AJOG, Samuel A. Cosgrove and Patricia A. Carter published "A Consideration of Therapeutic Abortion." On the one hand, they explicitly stated that "the deliberate and intentional interruption of fetal life and growth is actually murder. If this is so, then abortion is never justified more than any other murder is" (p. 303). Yet, "Is the murder which is abortion ever justifiable? The considered, honest opinion of many, probably a majority of medical practitioners of high scientific attainment and unimpeachable moral character, is yes!" (p. 304).

Cosgrove and Carter concluded that if abortion were sometimes justifiable, "it should be restricted in the same manner as is other 'justifiable' murder" (p. 304). At the same time, they noted, "There is a wide and increasing tendency to include in the evidence justifying abortion (a) remote threat to the mother's life, and hence (b) threat to the *health* of the mother. Thus Taussig repeatedly makes the plea for 'broader indications for therapeutic abortion.' Such broadening of indication for justifiable or 'therapeutic' feticide tends to practical removal of all deterrent to this practice" (ibid.).

Frederick Taussig would probably have strongly disagreed with the Cosgrove and Carter characterization of his views on abortion. After all, he had proposed several strategies for its prevention. The abortion controversy was nevertheless beginning to assume its contemporary shape, in which a "position"—pro-life or pro-choice—determines whether one believes a problem actually exists. Reducing Taussig's work to one "plea" not only misrepresented his views but also added to the confusion about the physician's medical responsibility.

The development of better and safer techniques of accomplishing abortion has contributed to the belief that the practitioner's medical responsibility is primarily a matter of the application of technical training. From the standpoint of epidemiological research, the technical problem centers on the incidence of morbidity and mortality associated with any procedure. In Taussig's opinion, the medical problem of abortion, in the context of the physician-patient relation, included more than the issue of whether it could be performed safely.

In the same article in which they criticized Taussig, Cosgrove and Carter provided a table detailing the "Incidence of Therapeutic Abortion in a Few Representative Clinics" (1944:305). The table showed that Johns Hopkins Hospital in 1941 had performed more therapeutic abortions than any other hospital in the country, one for every 35 deliveries. In a letter to AJOG in December 1944, Nicholson J. Eastman, head of the Department of Obstetrics at Johns Hopkins, reacted swiftly to the implied accusation. Eastman included his own table demonstrating that the Cosgrove and Carter figure distorted the Hopkins rate by focusing on a single year; for the years 1936 to 1944, Eastman estimated the rate to be one for every 65 deliveries (1944:892). Cosgrove's own institution, the Margaret Hague Maternity Hospital in Jersey City, New Jersey, appeared to have the lowest incidence of therapeutic abortions. This led Eastman to ask: "How in the world can one practice good obstetrics (and I do know that the practice of obstetrics at the Margaret Hague Maternity is excellent) with a therapeutic abortion rate of only 1 to 16,750 deliveries? If an incidence of 1 to 500 was cited, or even 1 to 1,000,

I would have regarded the report with envy and esteem, but 1 to 16,750 leaves me bewildered" (p. 893). Eastman concluded: "Can it possibly be that the views stated in this article [by Cosgrove and Carter], have been so thoroughly voiced in Jersey City over the years that cases requiring interruption are referred elsewhere?"(ibid.).

In his reply, included in the same issue, Cosgrove insisted that "there was no invidious purpose in having picked out a particular year which showed this incidence of therapeutic abortions [at Hopkins] especially high" (1944:893). In response to Eastman's suggestion that his hospital's low rate was the result of referrals to other hospitals, he acknowledged the existence of "two unrecognized hospitals in this area, both small, where the incidence of abortion might well be in higher ratio than is consistent with any standard of good practice." However, he claimed, these hospitals "are not attended by such men of good conscience as we like to think of ourselves being, and therefore, the work done therein would be quite beyond the pale of our discussion" (p. 894). Cosgrove passed back the referral "accusation" to Eastman: "The graduates of Johns Hopkins look to it for help in their own problems, and refer their own difficulties for solution on a relatively tremendous scale" (p. 895).

Referral appeared to play an important part in the medical management of abortion. A physician's prerogative to refer a patient was also the privilege of avoiding potentially controversial cases. On the other hand, a physician's willingness to perform an abortion was influenced by the training environment and the kinds of medical expertise available. The debate between Eastman and Cosgrove touched upon issues in the practice of obstetrics and gynecology that transcended the religious differences between practitioners. Both men argued about the principles and practice of medicine.

Years later, in 1953, Eastman recalled the Cosgrove and Carter article in an editor's note in *Obstetrical and Gynecological Survey*. Once again, as in his letter to the editor of AJOG in 1944, Eastman sought to clarify "something of a sampling error" associated with the Cosgrove and Carter report of Johns Hopkins' record on this matter (1953:219). He reflected further:

The paramount aim of obstetrics is the preservation of maternal life and health; and therapeutic abortion must find its sole justification (if it can be justified) in the degree to which it serves that end. The incidence of therapeutic interruption of pregnancy in any given clinic or state, while informative, is not the main issue; the real question is: Do all these operations actually spare mothers' lives?

We used to think so in our clinic, as our record shows, but over the years a goodly number of patients have refused the operative intervention which we recommended and from these brave women (or stubborn, senseless women, as you would have it) we have learned more about the true indications for therapeutic abortion than from all the articles that have been written on the subject. Yes, every Christmas I receive a little photograph of a certain Mrs. P. and her small daughter, who is now five years old. When Mrs. P. first came to us, about 20 weeks pregnant with that little girl, and objected adamantly to therapeutic abortion, we considered her as good as dead right then and there, because she had the worst case of rheumatic heart disease that ever was. She had all the bad signs: age of 35 and a history of repeated attacks of decompensation. In fact, during the previous year she had learned to feel as much at home in an oxygen tent as out of it. The remainder of the pregnancy she spent in our hospital in bed, in and out of failure; and as the last straw, she went beyond term with a big baby presenting by the breech and premature rupture of the membranes. Nevertheless, she was delivered vaginally and, as already stated, for five years now she has sent me a nice little photograph each Christmas showing herself and her daughter out in their vegetable garden. I sometimes wonder if the regularity with which she sends these cards is not based in part on a desire to pull my leg a little about the therapeutic abortion which I recommended and she refused. (1953:220)

Eastman argued that the incidence of therapeutic abortion in hospitals across the country revealed little about what he took the central issue to be: Was maternal mortality reduced by the resort to therapeutic abortion? Curiously, instead of calling for more epidemiological studies of the sort used by Carter and Cosgrove to criticize Johns Hopkins, he recited an anecdote about his experience with one patient.

Eastman's 1953 comment contained a reluctant criticism of medical common sense. Although Carter and Cosgrove had argued from the premise that abortion was rarely justified, their statistics did not necessarily prove that a broadening of medical indications for abortion was the cause of the higher incidence of the procedure at Johns Hopkins. Eastman's anecdote suggested that the rate might very well have been higher but for the tenacity of certain patients in refusing the recommendation of their doctors.

It has become a truism to propose that any abortion is safer for the mother than delivering a full-term infant. If one were to devise an abortion policy solely on this epidemiological conclusion, it would follow that no pregnancy should be brought to term. The absurdity of such a policy can be understood only in a context quite different from the epidemiological one. Eastman's anecdote about Mrs. P. revealed that medical common sense relied on more than statistical probabilities; it was also influenced by the specific interaction between a patient and a physician—and in this case, by the patient's willingness to risk her life to bring her pregnancy to term.

Since Taussig's time the range of medical indications for the interruption of pregnancy has sharply declined. Now the physician is expected to consider the mental health aspects of the meaning of *medical* or to redefine the interest of the patient in such a way that she is permitted to interrupt a pregnancy (with the aid of a medically licensed practitioner) whenever she elects. In one sense the broadening of medical indications for abortion represents a further medicalization of the procedure; in another sense, the patient's right to elect the procedure for any reason whatsoever represents its complete demedicalization. [5] When linked with the *preservation* of life, abortion was construed as an instance of medical failure. When linked with the safe *termination* of an early pregnancy, it lost its status as a last resort and became a relatively simple surgical procedure. Its complex medical legacy would nevertheless persist in the minds of some practitioners.

With a greater uncertainty during the 1950s about what constituted true medical indications for therapeutic abortion, the medical profession relied increasingly on decision by committee to underscore the medical consensus for each procedure performed. Therapeutic abortion committees often consisted of physicians from several specialties, including internal medicine, obstetrics and gynecology, and psychiatry. In some cases, the committees included hospital administrators and other nonmedical representatives. In retrospect, Kristin Luker has argued, these committees were more a delaying tactic than a resolution among physicians about how best to determine when an abortion was indicated (1984b:56). Psychiatry, in particular, played an influential part in the diagnosis of indications, thus gradually confining the role of the ob/gyn to the technical task of performing the procedure as safely as possible. [6]

From the mid-1940s until well into the 1960s, the indications for therapeutic abortion and the role of therapeutic abortion committees were discussed and debated in the obstetric and gynecologic litera-ture.[7] The committees were supposed to provide a more objective basis for evaluating the therapeutic purposes of each procedure. They undoubtedly relieved many practitioners of the responsibility for having to underwrite the medical necessity for abortion. During this time a noticeable reduction in the performance of abortions occurred in some hospitals, though by no means in all of them (Grisez, 1970:96–100).

Psychiatric indications for therapeutic abortion were not easily adapted to the practice of obstetrics and gynecology. Deeply com-mitted to the successful management of pregnancy, obstetrician/ gynecologists were reluctant to accept the idea that abortion was indicated except in dire circumstances. If abortion was to be heralded as a right, this was in part due to a change in attitude among medical professionals in general about the purpose of the procedure. Efforts leading to the liberalization of abortion laws in some states and even-tually to the Supreme Court rulings in 1973 were certainly strength-ened by the testimony of physicians who called for an easing of restrictions (Steinhoff and Diamond, 1977).

Until more was known about the prenatal diagnosis of genetic abnormalities and the effects of certain drugs upon fetal development, abortion remained a subject for medical rather than public debate. Focus on the health of the unborn initiated a reassessment of the indications for abortion during the 1960s (Nadler, 1971). Clinical research aimed at preserving the lives of both mother and child con-tinued and advanced, but physicians' acceptance of abortion as a form of elective surgery had yet to be reconciled with an understanding of their medical responsibilities.

2
The Physician in the Abortion Controversy

The debate over physician responsibility for abortion increasingly took place outside the profession during the 1950s and 1960s as the inconsistencies in state laws prohibiting it were challenged. The increasing availability of abortion throughout the world was regarded, especially among the upper classes, as evidence of the need to accept it as a legitimate part of family planning. The proliferation of opinion polls taken of physicians' attitudes about abortion presented a new image of the profession to the general public. Doctors no longer appeared to be united about the medical indications for the procedure. Their professional uncertainty opened the way for a probing of public opinion.

During this time pharmaceutical companies began to introduce new forms of contraception. With the rise of the women's movement, the right to birth control encompassed a broad range of new expectations about the relationships between women and men, husbands and wives, patients and doctors, and parents and children.[1] Abortion was viewed less as a failure in family planning than as a necessary factor in personal and economic liberation. The decision to have or not to have children no longer depended on whether one chose to have sexual relations or on the imperfect technologies of contraception.

Epidemiological studies of the morbidity and mortality associated with legalized induced abortion all but replaced the previous sixty years of medical discussion about how the practice might be discouraged. Such studies were conducted, for example, in Eastern Europe, Scandinavia, and Japan (Potts *et al.*, 1977; David *et al.*, 1978; Coleman, 1983). Improved knowledge about the relative safety of induced abortion around the world led to greater scrutiny of American medical practice.

At the June 1967 meeting of the American Medical Association in Atlantic City, New Jersey, the Committee on Human Reproduction submitted a detailed report and policy recommendation on therapeutic abortion that was actually a response to and a "modification of the Model Penal Code of the American Law Institute" (*Journal of the American Medical Association,* 1967). The Model Penal Code had been proposed eight years earlier by the American Law Institute, and the section on "Abortion and Related Offenses" made ample reference to Frederick Taussig's *Abortion, Spontaneous and Induced* (1936) when giving figures on the incidence of criminal abortion in America (American Law Institute, 1959:146–166). The code included the following indications for justified abortion: life-threatening impairment to the physical or mental health of the mother, grave physical or mental defect in the unborn, and pregnancy as a result of rape, incest, or other felonious intercourse (Sloane and Horvitz, 1973:134–135).

Two factors contributed to the medical profession's reluctance to respond quickly to these proposed indications. On the one hand, the laws prohibiting abortion in the nineteenth century, as noted in chapter 1, received the strong support of a profession seeking to define and control the conditions under which the procedure could be performed. On the other hand, modification of the nineteenth-century laws had already begun in many states without the official endorsement of the AMA. Legislative initiatives to rewrite state laws followed major outbreaks of rubella and the thalidomide tragedy during the early 1960s (Luker, 1984b). Christopher Tietze has pointed out that "in 1964, about 4000 abortions were performed because the pregnant woman had contracted rubella during the first trimester of pregnancy, although this type of indication was then not recognized by the statutes of any state" (1976:2).

When the Supreme Court ruled in 1973 on two separate abortion cases (*Roe v. Wade* and *Doe v. Bolton*), the legacy of professional solidarity finally came to an end. In *Roe v. Wade*, the Court established a woman's constitutional right to the procedure, although it acknowledged that this right was not absolute. In other words, a woman's right to an abortion did not compel a physician to perform the operation and could be exercised only until the time of viability, or that time when the fetus/infant is supposed to be able to live independently of the mother. If professional solidarity had ever existed about the medical indications for abortion and about how the medical decision to perform one should be made, both court cases in effect diminished the importance of medical thinking for deciding how to proceed. The medical profession's attempt in the nineteenth century to write medical conduct into the law was thus overturned.

The Court acknowledged that medical knowledge, not legal principle, played a crucial role in its assessment of the differences between 1873 and 1973. In *Doe v. Bolton*, a case that addressed the constitutionality of abortion statutes in Georgia, the Court noted:

> The appellants recognize that a century ago medical knowledge was not so advanced as it is today, that the techniques of antisepsis were not known, and that any abortion procedure was dangerous for the woman. To restrict the legality of the abortion to the situation where it was deemed necessary, in medical judgment, for the preservation of the woman's life was only a natural conclusion in the exercise of the legislative judgment of that time (see Walbert and Butler, 1973:369; the full texts of both decisions are reprinted there, along with relevant parts of state statutes and of the Model Penal Code).[2]

Doe v. Bolton also held that therapeutic abortion committees were unconstitutional. Both women and doctors were freer to decide what to do within the limits established by both cases. In this sense, the Court's rulings were a victory not only for those seeking greater reproductive freedom but also for physicians seeking the right to determine when they would participate in abortion or, for that matter, any elective surgery. It should not be surprising (as will be seen) that the abandonment of medical indications for abortion and the dismantling of therapeutic abortion committees led to an enormous transformation in the delivery of abortion services in the United States. For women obtaining abortions today, the matters of accessibility and expense have replaced the earlier struggles to undo the legacy of medical indications and decision by committee. The consequences of the Court's rulings for physicians have received far less public attention. This is due in part to the fact that, after the Supreme Court rulings in 1973, abortion became a national dilemma. When the Court ruled that abortion was a private matter between physician and patient and that it could be restricted only to safeguard the health of the pregnant woman, the political forces for and against these changes were set in motion.

Physician and public opinion on abortion should not be interpreted apart from both changing social expectations and advancing medical knowledge. In 1949, sociologists David Riesman and Nathan Glazer concluded:

> The scientific study of public opinion is thus today in the hands of neither the poll-takers nor the respondents: both are caught in an historical process which has not only set the questions to be investigated but also the form of the answer. We should at least assume that another structure of opinion may exist, in which every question has many sides, and many perspectives in which it may be viewed, each tinged with varying degrees of meaning and affect. (1954:494)

An example of this historical process can be found in the Louis Harris polls taken of public attitudes toward abortion. Twice during 1972, respondents were asked: "Do you favor or oppose allowing legalized abortions to take place up to *four months* [italics added] of pregnancy?" (1976a:265). Nationally, public opinion was virtually evenly divided on the question. In June 1972, 48 percent favored, 43 percent opposed, and 9 percent were not sure. In August 1972, 42 percent favored, 46 percent opposed, and 12 percent were not sure.

Following the Supreme Court rulings of January 1973, another poll was conducted, this time in the language that the Court used in its decisions:

> The U.S. Supreme Court recently decided that state laws which make it illegal for a woman to have an abortion are unconstitutional, and that the decision on whether a woman should have an abortion up to three months' pregnancy should be left to a woman and her doctor to decide. In general, do you favor or oppose the U.S. Supreme Court decision making abortions up to three months' pregnancy legal? (1976b:387)

The nationwide poll of February 1973 indicated that 52 percent favored the Court decision, 41 percent opposed it, and 7 percent were not sure. The Harris pollsters, in less than a year, changed the length of gestation of pregnancy from four months to three months in their question in direct response to the Supreme Court's division of pregnancy into three trimesters. The Court proposed this trimester view of pregnancy in order to give guidelines for what was required of the medical profession and the state, especially in the second and third trimesters.

Public opinion and Court opinion are difficult to disentangle insofar as the public response is constructed within the framework of the Court's rulings. The February 1973 poll was just as indicative of public approval and disapproval of the Court's intervention in the abortion issue as it was of public opinion about when one should be permitted to interrupt pregnancy. Public opinion polls did not address what types of techniques should be used for abortion or how far along in a pregnancy a right existed to interrupt it.

The Court took for granted that medical knowledge about physiological growth was sufficient to define *viability*, or that point in gestation when the fetus/infant could survive outside the uterus (around twenty-eight weeks at that time). The pollsters, however unwittingly, acknowledged the authority of medical knowledge by not pursuing the general public's definition of viability. Many physicians, faced with the practical realities of improved medical technology, would be less inclined to rely on legal and public opinion as guides to how they should act.

In their global study of the medical and social dimensions of abortion practice, Malcolm Potts, Peter Diggory, and John Peel observed that in the United States, "at the point when the changes became most rapid, a number of surveys of doctors' opinions were conducted; indeed the sudden multiplication of surveys in 1967 was about as sensitive a marker of change as the content of the surveys themselves" (Potts *et al.*, 1977:358). In 1974, Emily Campbell Moore-Cavar prepared the *International Inventory of Information on Induced Abortion*, which included more than six hundred pages of synopses of the religious, ethical, legal, medical, psychological, administrative, and demographic aspects of abortion.

Moore-Cavar listed twenty-three surveys (one of which was a

combined survey taken in Canada and the United States) of physician opinion about abortion taken between 1965 and 1973. Of the twenty-three surveys, eight were devoted entirely to ascertaining the opinions of obstetrician/gynecologists, who presumably would be most likely to be called upon to perform abortions. There were few surprises in the breakdown according to religion: Catholic practitioners generally opposed changes in the laws prohibiting abortion, and Jewish and Protestant practitioners generally approved of the liberalization or complete abolition of the prohibition.

Prior to 1973, most of the surveys asked for physicians' opinions on their respective state laws. In many surveys a list of different medical and social circumstances that would indicate or justify abortion was presented. Respondents rated each circumstance with either approval or disapproval. There is considerable evidence that "elective" or patient-requested abortions were the least approved among doctors, whereas few had difficulty giving unqualified approval for an abortion when a woman's life was endangered.

For example, in a 1969 issue of *Modern Medicine,* a free medical newsletter with a circulation of approximately two hundred thousand, 27,741 physicians replied to the question "Should abortion be available to any woman capable of giving legal consent upon her own request to a competent physician?" (Modern Medicine, 1969:19). Unqualified approval was lowest among physicians in general practice (39%), followed by ob/gyns (41%) and general surgeons (45%). Highest approval came from plastic surgeons (73%), followed by psychiatrists (72%) and allergists (64%). In a survey taken of members of the Georgia Medical Association in 1970, only 25 percent of the obstetrician/gynecologists who responded approved of abortion on request. This was in contrast to 66 percent approval by psychiatrists (Freeman and Graves, 1970).

The specialty of obstetrics and gynecology in these survey data represented the profession's most conservative attitude toward abortion; psychiatry represented the most liberal. Psychiatrists, allergists, and plastic surgeons are, however, least likely to perform abortions and no doubt less likely than obstetrician/gynecologists to be asked to perform them. Pollsters were uninterested in the distinction between who would approve and who would perform.

The problem of physician opinion is further complicated if one examines how patient populations perceive physician participation in abortion and family planning services. Era L. Hill and Johan W. Eliot observed in their 1972 study "Black Physicians' Experience with Abortion Requests and Opinion About Abortion Law Change in Michigan":

> [The] perception of benefit to black women does not mean that members of the Detroit Medical Society were insensitive to charges of "genocide" leveled by some black leaders against family planning programs, particularly those programs that label black women and poor women as "target populations." It does mean simply that along with their clear recognition of undesirable motivations on the part of some proponents of family planning, they also recognize the overriding need of black and indigent women for medically safe family planning and abortion services, for protection of their health and family life (1972:57).

The political role of family planning services in achieving a better life for the poor has centered on the degree to which such services are perceived to be either a social improvement or a social necessity. Abortion has come to symbolize this difference insofar as funding for it and other forms of birth control is seen as an efficient means for reducing the number of people in the world. The freedom to choose abortion should not be separated from the claim made by many that greater efforts must be made to preserve the world's finite resources.

In a 1970 survey, 67 members of the Johns Hopkins Department of Obstetrics and Gynecology were asked about their willingness to perform abortions of pregnancies of twelve weeks or less and twelve weeks or more (Wolf *et al.*, 1971:141–47). Of the 53 who replied, 10 said that they would not perform abortions for any reason. These ten included four house staff members who had not completed residency, three full-time and attending staff members who had completed residency prior to 1961, and three full-time and attending staff members who had completed residency after 1960. The survey investigators wrote of the ten: "We felt that physicians morally opposed to and unwilling to perform abortion for any reason had deeply ingrained attitudes formed independently of their educational process (which is our concern here) and not likely to be changed by it" (Wolf *et al.*, 1971:144).

Of the 43 remaining physicians, all 15 house staff who had not completed residency were willing to perform abortions before or after twelve weeks. Of the 13 full-time and attending staff members who had completed residency after 1960, 12 were willing to perform abortions before twelve weeks and 11 after twelve weeks. Of the 15 full-time and attending staff members who had completed residency before 1961, 11 would perform abortions before twelve weeks and 8 after twelve weeks. These data suggest that older staff members were more reluctant to perform abortions, especially later in pregnancy. Perhaps the trend toward a greater willingness to perform abortions followed generational lines; the older practitioners approved less and the younger ones approved more.

But this conclusion does not address the status differences among physicians in the training hierarchy of Johns Hopkins or any other residency program. Given the rapid changes in law that occurred between 1967 and 1973, the rising demand for abortions (along with a decline in the birth rate) contributed to a greater willingness on the part of ob/gyns to perform them. Of course every resident in obstetrics and gynecology is expected to know how to perform a dilation and curettage, if only to be able to treat an incomplete abortion. The new expectation that younger practitioners should be thoroughly familiar with abortion techniques undoubtedly had consequences for how clinical work was assigned (Hall, 1971; Kopelman and Douglas, 1971; Stone et al., 1971).

Six months after the Johns Hopkins study was reported, the *American Journal of Obstetrics and Gynecology* published the findings of a study entitled "Therapeutic Abortion: Attitudes of Medical Personnel Leading to Complications in Patient Care." The authors reviewed medical records of fifty patients who had received therapeutic abortions at Presbyterian-St. Luke's Hospital in Chicago. For the same study, the authors held ten seminars in order to research the psychological aspects of obstetrics and gynecology with particular attention to therapeutic abortion. They found that

> residents more often avoid their assignment to participate with curettages and therapeutic abortions than with vaginal hysterectomies. . . . Negative feelings toward a therapeutic abortion are frequently expressed in the seminars and corridors by experienced gynecologists and trainees alike. . . . Several surgeons attempt to rationalize that their feelings do not arise out

of the problem of life and death, citing various arguments as to the onset of life. *We submit that in spite of the physician's studied rationalizations, the reason for avoidance of the surgery is concern with the issue of causing a death.* The pressures of society toward a large increase in the number of therapeutic abortions may find us unequipped to meet our responsibility. Those who do perform the abortion or assist in the procedure must not only perfect their technique but also must resolve their own understandably ambivalent feelings. (Wolff *et al.*, 1971:732–733, footnotes omitted)

Conducted two years before the Supreme Court rulings, the Johns Hopkins and Presbyterian-St. Luke studies suggested a developing split in the professional view of the aims of obstetrical and gynecological work. Both studies could have been used to support the political positions of pro-choice or pro-life, but instead of reflecting the politicization of those who devised them, they were a response to the real increase in demand for abortions made upon the medical profession. (See also Mascovich *et al.*, 1973.)

A pilot study of the sources of Connecticut physicians' attitudes toward abortion, published in the *American Journal of Public Health* in 1976, concluded that "religion, early experiences within the family of orientation and the physician's family of procreation—that is, those areas of life which are the most personal and most intimate—are judged by these physicians as being far more important than the broad range of professional experiences which occur later in life" (Pratt *et al.*, 1976:289). The authors further observed:

[The] variables of age, date of completion of medical school, board certification, percentage of time in obstetrics and gynecology, geographic location of the medical school from which the physician received his degree, and the size of the community in which the physician's office is located (urban vs. rural) are not significantly related to attitudes toward abortion among this sample of physicians. (ibid.)

The variables constructed to assess "professional experiences" in this pilot study do not adequately address the changing character of those experiences in light of the legalization of abortion. It is how, not whether, abortion has been accommodated to the practice of medicine that remains to be considered.

The fact that most people today have an opinion about abortion demonstrates how the question of its rightness or wrongness pervades the collective conscience of America. But opinions of individuals, when measured for the purpose of describing what the "typical" American believes about the matter, are thoroughly dependent on what questions are asked and, as Judith Blake has shown, in what form they are asked (1971:540–549; see also Blake and Pinal, 1981:309–320). The physician's role takes on added importance because the abortion decision is made not only by the woman requesting the procedure. A physician's refusal to perform an abortion is probably of less consequence than a woman's inability to obtain one, but this emphasis conceals how abortion services are delivered in American society. Opinion polls may indicate a public willingness to tolerate abortion as well as a willingness on the part of the medical profession to permit abortion, but the specialty that has assumed the responsibility for providing the service has not easily accommodated it to the practice of medicine. The abortion clinic, either freestanding or hospital-affiliated, symbolizes this lack of accommodation.

In the April 1, 1972, issue of the *American Journal of Obstetrics and Gynecology,* one hundred professors of obstetrics and gynecology signed a public statement that was intended to be a response to the impending changes in American abortion law and practice. All those who signed were full professors at their respective medical schools; fifty-eight were chairmen or heads of departments of obstetrics and gynecology. Their statement was extraordinary in several respects. Although it was not supposed to reflect the sentiments of any particular medical society or of the American College of Obstetricians and Gynecologists, it did embody the authoritative opinion of the teaching wing of the profession.

The professors conceded in the opening paragraphs that times were changing:

> Many physicians still believe that abortions should be done only for medical reasons and that only they are qualified to determine when these reasons exist. In order to comply with the new laws and court decisions, however, it will be necessary for physicians to realize that abortion has become a predominately social as well as medical responsibility. For the first time, except perhaps for cosmetic surgery, doctors will be expected to do an operation simply because the patient asks that it be done. Granted, this changes the physician's traditional role, but it will be necessary to make this change if we are to serve the new society in which we live. ("A Statement on Abortion by One Hundred Professors of Obstetrics," 1972:992)

The professors contended that abortions would have to be made available to rich and poor alike. They proposed no specific measures for how the profession should organize to provide such services to all who requested them. But they considered it their moral responsibility to point out the inequities in access to abortions in private facilities. Their manifesto was, in this respect, an acknowledgment of other inequities in the provision of medical resources that appeared to call for further concessions on the part of the profession to serve the "new society in which we live."[3]

Suspicious of government regulation and unaccustomed to liberation movements among patients, the medical profession has appeared to be conservative, on the defensive, and in an endless confrontation with courts and social movements supporting or opposing access to abortion. The professors' insistence that the profession must *serve* rather than *lead* the new society lent further support to this inference. That the teaching cadre of obstetrics and gynecology was the first part of the specialty to resign itself to the new society marked a profound transformation in professional attitudes about what counted as the best medical care.

The professors realized that doctors would be besieged with requests for the procedure as the result of changes in the abortion laws: "The doctor with conscientious objections must, of course, be excused, but he will be expected to refer his patients elsewhere" (1972:992). In this seemingly unconscious recognition of the political wars about to follow the complete legalization of abortion, the professors warned that conscientious objection would have to be consistent: "A more difficult dilemma will be faced by the doctor who approves of abortions for some reasons but not all, for he may be accused of being unduly arbitrary or capricious" (ibid.).

They advised hospital administrators that "although there is no medical contraindication to admitting clean abortion cases to a maternity floor, there are obvious psychological advantages to segregating these cases" (p. 993). Here was an instance of an institutional splitting brought about not by the conservatism of the traditional health care system but rather by those who were faced with performing what they believed was a very different kind of medical work alongside obstetrical deliveries. The charge of conservatism against the profession may appear to explain why abortions are performed less often within the traditional health care system than within the system of freestanding clinics (see Nathanson and Becker, 1981). But how do those who make this charge explain why abortion clinics are less inclined than obstetrician/gynecologists in private practice to offer prenatal services? The division of obstetric and gynecologic work calls for a more systematic treatment of physician social psychology and of the social psychology of institutions.

An appeal to medical indications for abortion was contained in the professors' statement, even though they conceded the overwhelming impact of social indications:

> It should be emphasized that abortion is medically defined as the termination of pregnancy before the end of the twentieth week. Regardless of the wording of a particular state law, therefore, abortions should not be performed for purely social reasons beyond this gestational age. Every effort should be made, of course, to perform abortions before the end of the first trimester. (1972:993)

This odd recommendation followed an earlier insistence that a physician's role in performing an abortion should be viewed primarily as a social responsibility. Why a "purely social" reason was any less legitimate after the twentieth week than before was explained by how an abortion is "medically defined." The 1973 Supreme Court rulings, permitting abortion for any reason until the time of "viability," would point to the inappropriateness of drawing lines in this way.

Because abortion on request was still regarded as a last resort, the professors noted that "sterilization will play a role in curtailing recidivism." Yet, they carefully advised: "Approval of an abortion request, on the other hand, should not be conditional upon the applicant's submission to sterilization." Perhaps in recognition of the fact that they were opening the way for abortion as a routine form of birth control, they concluded:

> An integral part of any abortion program should be postoperative provision of contraceptive advice. Although women should be relieved, insofar as possible, of any sense of shame or guilt from the abortion experience, they should not be encouraged to regard abortion as a primary method of birth control. (1972:994)

As for the legacy of the American birth-control movement and of the many decades of medical concern about abortion, the crucial contrast between that time and ours may lie in the professors' use of the word *primary*. The intention of family planners was to reduce the need for abortion. This is not to say that there would ever come a time when abortion practice disappeared completely. The professors' insistence that it should not be a *primary* method of birth control confirmed a change in attitude and belief about the future of birth control in America.

In 1970, Governor Nelson Rockefeller signed into law the New York State Abortion Statute, which permitted abortions to be performed for any reason during the first two trimesters of pregnancy. Dr. Bernard N. Nathanson, a practicing obstetrician/gynecologist, assumed a major role in the formation of abortion clinics during that time. In the *New England Journal of Medicine* in November 1974, Nathanson recounted his participation in the effort to legalize abortion in New York State:

> Our next goal was to assure ourselves that low cost, safe and humane abortions were available to all, and to that end we established the Center for Reproductive and Sexual Health, which was the first—and largest—abortion clinic in the Western world. (1974:1189)[4]

After a year and a half as director of the center, Nathanson resigned, explaining that "the Center had performed 60,000 abortions with no maternal deaths—an outstanding record of which we are proud. However, I am deeply troubled by my own increasing certainty that I had in fact presided over 60,000 deaths" (1974:1189). Repeating the insights of several generations of obstetrician/gynecologists before him, Nathanson asserted: "There is no longer serious doubt in my mind that human life exists within the womb from the very onset of pregnancy, despite the fact that the nature of the intrauterine life has been the subject of considerable dispute in the past" (ibid.).

Nathanson directed his confession to those who performed abortions. His "increasing certainty" about his role was then followed by an obvious denial of the physician's culpability:

> Certainly, the medical profession itself cannot shoulder the burden of this matter. The phrase "between a woman and her physician" is an empty one since the physician is only the instrument of her decision, and has no special knowledge of the moral dilemma or the ethical agony involved in the decision. Furthermore, there are seldom any purely medical indi-

cations for abortion. The decision is the most serious responsibility a woman can experience in her lifetime, and at present it is hers alone. (1974:1189)

This unambiguous depiction of who bears the burden of moral responsibility undermines any presumption of physician authority over the decision and confirms an image of the physician as only a technical means to ends determined entirely by patients. But Nathanson's own stated reasons for moving against unproscribed abortion suggest that an "ethical agony" may exist for doctors as much as for women. As "only the instrument of her decision," the physician is not expected to ask for or judge the reasons for the abortion. This is, finally, what is meant by a constitutionally protected right to privacy.[5]

In later writings, Dr. Nathanson moved more decidedly into the camp persuaded against abortion.[6] His approach to those who defended abortion but who, unlike himself, had never actively participated in the culture of abortion clinics was to analyze various arguments advanced by contemporary philosophers and bioethicists. The turn to ethical analysis was also an acceptance of the subordinate role of medical thinking in general. A more rational and emotionally removed analysis of the problem, he hoped, would help transform the culture of abortion clinics across the country. He did not seek solutions in either law or pedagogy, as Frederick Taussig had done many decades before. Instead, he insisted on careful assessment of philosophical arguments which proposed, for instance, that women "rise at least to the level of Judith Thomson's Minimally Decent Samaritan" (Nathanson and Ostling, 1979:231).[7]

The distance between Taussig's strategies for preventing abortion and Nathanson's philosophy of Samaritanism confirms a real change in attitude about the prospects for reducing the resort to abortion. Before the promulgation of philosophical and ethical analyses about the right to life and the right to choose, physicians had already adapted to a narrower view of their responsibilities toward the procedure. They are now expected to assess its technical aspects: efficiency, safety, and access form the new moral vocabulary of the epidemiology of abortion. To moralize about patient behavior and responsibility is interpreted as "professional dominance." An individualistic ethic and a preoccupation with the statistics of risk are the bases of the new view of professional responsibility, equally moralistic as the earlier attempts to write physician conduct about abortion into the law but better suited for a time when the privilege to prescribe is linked with "informed consent" rather than with patient "compliance."

Both epidemiology and ethics are assigned higher social prestige and influence than are specific programs intended to reduce the resort to abortion. The character of this prestige is important to remark on sociologically. The social role of philosophers and ethicists on government commissions who deliberate bioethical issues such as abortion must be compared to the now publicly acknowledged failure of family planning programs to reduce the demand for this form of birth control, for which there is believed to be a better alternative. The goals of bioethics differ from the educational tasks of social work (Callahan, 1983) and also reflect a disdain for the nonrational authority of social movements (on either side of the issue) that have opposed and threaten to supplant the incremental logic of social policy advisers. At the same time, this "value-free" movement has come to dominate governmental and intellectual discussions about the identification of social problems in American society (Fox and Swazey, 1984).

In the West, a tradition of special permissions for abortion was once embodied in religious casuistries and medical judgments. The contemporary philosopher-ethicist who in principle wishes to defend liberal and pluralist culture does not appeal to these traditions as authoritative except to exercise reason against them.[8] The appeal, with rare exception, is made to an academic discourse in philosophy whose range includes Kantian, liberal-utilitarian, and libertarian voices. Categorical arguments explore the nature of "person" and "personhood." Liberal-utilitarian arguments focus more specifically on the circumstances in which abortion should be permitted. Libertarian arguments assess the rights that pertain to all involved. The three perspectives no doubt overlap, but each depicts a fundamental philosophical approach to contemporary thinking about abortion.[9] The physician's decision to perform the procedure is guided by principles that are less rooted in this form of intellectual life and more pervasive in medical practice itself. That these principles of practice persist despite the ascension of bioethics points to the widening space between the day-to-day practice of medicine in this matter and the proliferation of intellectual debates about when abortion is justified.

The ethical approach, to which Nathanson subscribes and to which he attaches great hope, focuses on changes that will not be reversed simply by rational argument. With the legal and medical status of abortion so fundamentally altered by judicial mandate, ethical analyses have probed the conditions of choice by and large from the perspective of the woman submitting to the procedure. Yet those who are asked to perform it have raised and continue to raise questions about their responsibilities.

Unlike Bernard Nathanson, Frederick Taussig believed that abortion was a special medical responsibility. Ethical perspectives have taken for granted the relative safety of an abortion performed early in pregnancy and have rejected the physician's authority over the procedure, except in its seemingly technical aspects. Efforts to discourage the practice, either in law or through pedagogy, are no longer the distinctive responsibility of medical practitioners. The delivery of abortion services in America has nevertheless continued to implicate the medical profession, whose search for its proper role depends on far more than an ethics of choice.

3
Medical Practice and Family Planning in Daleton

The confrontations that shape the politics of birth control at the national level dissolve in the face of the day-to-day medical practices of doctors, who remain the sole legal providers of abortion and other forms of birth control. Obstetrician/gynecologists assume the primary surgical and medical responsibilities for such procedures as sexual sterilization and abortion and for the prescription of diaphragms, IUDs (intrauterine devices), and oral contraceptives.

Whether for reasons of safety, efficiency, or convenience, the modern development of birth control has increased the participation of professionals, including physicians, research scientists, and social workers, in the monitoring and controlling of birth (Arney, 1982). In what follows, I offer several explanations for why birth control services, despite their medicalization, exist on the fringes of physician care and responsibility. The provision of these services by large-scale clinics calls for a better understanding of the other medical context in which they are offered, namely, the private practice of medicine.

The Community of Daleton

"Daleton" is a moderate-sized city (approximately 100,000) located in the northeastern United States. It is the county seat for "Shireton" County, which has a population of nearly

37

300,000. The community of Daleton supports three hospitals, which serve the greater part of the county and to a lesser extent the rural parts of adjacent counties. Other major hospital centers are between thirty and fifty miles away.

Daleton Hospital, the oldest and largest, is the only one with residency training. Programs are offered in internal medicine, family practice, obstetrics/gynecology, radiology, anesthesiology, pathology, surgery, and psychiatry. It has a staff of more than 200 physicians and 40 residents, and beds for over 600 patients.

The two other hospitals, St. Timothy and Central Hospital, do not compare in physical plant to Daleton Hospital, but each has expanded its services to the community over the years. St. Timothy, a Catholic hospital, is a little more than half the size of Daleton Hospital, with 330 beds and 130 on the medical staff. In contrast to Daleton Hospital, which is adjacent to the wealthiest part of the metropolitan area, St. Timothy is located in Daleton's Polish and Italian working-class neighborhoods. Central Hospital is the smallest of the three hospitals, with approximately 200 beds and 80 on its medical staff. It is located in the center of Daleton, where private residences are mixed with professional offices of lawyers, physicians, and dentists.

The Community of Practitioners

Of the twenty-six obstetrician/gynecologists who practiced in Daleton during the time that interviews were conducted, only one refused to be interviewed; another was willing to talk only briefly by telephone.[1] The others agreed to be interviewed in their offices, at hospitals, or at home. Nearly half of these doctors had done part or all of their specialty training at Daleton Hospital. This training consisted of four years of hospital work (one year as an intern, three years as a resident) after completion of medical school. The average age of an obstetrician/gynecologist beginning in private practice in Daleton was thirty years old.[2]

Six group practices specializing in obstetrics and gynecology on a fee-for-service basis operated in Daleton. Four of those six were affiliated with Daleton Hospital, and they accounted for fourteen of the twenty-six ob/gyns (see fig. 3.1). Of the two remaining groups (with two members in each), one was affiliated with St. Timothy

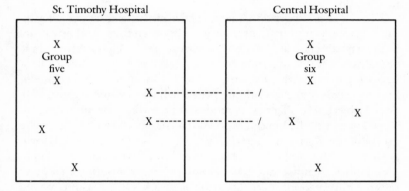

Figure 3.1 Hospital Affiliations of Obstetrician/Gynecologists in Daleton.

and the other with Central. Only one solo practitioner was on staff at Daleton Hospital; four were on staff at St. Timothy and three at Central.

At a time of increased specialization within medicine, it was not surprising to find more physicians practicing in groups. One of the younger doctors who belonged to a group remarked: "Obstetrics is one of the worst specialties to build up a practice in. You don't have many deliveries in your first few months of private practice because your first patients don't come to you about to give birth—they've gone elsewhere months before." Besides reducing the individual practitioner's overhead, a group practice enables one colleague to fill in for another. Benefits for the practitioner include the opportunity to coordinate daily work schedules and vacations more regularly. The physician in group practice can also specialize with the understanding that his colleagues will refer cases to him.

Family Planning in Daleton

For many years, Planned Parenthood in Daleton received much of its support from United Way funds. Its clinic offered routine contraceptive information as well as medical examinations by physicians drawn from the resident staff of Daleton Hospital. Neither abortion services nor abortion referrals were provided by Planned Parenthood in Daleton.

There was no abortion clinic in Daleton. In fact, clinics offering this service on an outpatient basis were between thirty and fifty miles away. The absence of abortion services at the family planning clinic in Daleton was due in part to public protests made by Catholic members of United Way's Executive Board. One physician explained: "Several years ago the Catholic priests who sit on the United Way Board objected to Planned Parenthood providing abortion services. They apparently had enough power to cut off all the funds, so the group doing abortion referrals within Planned Parenthood, known as Choice, was thrown out. Choice now literally operates out of people's homes." Choice is a national volunteer organization that gives referral information about abortion services. On occasion, young women, mostly teenagers with no regular private physician, were referred to Choice by the staff of Daleton's Planned Parenthood clinic. Counselors working for Choice often referred their clients to the clinics outside the community.

With the availability of abortion services an hour away, Daleton physicians and family planning advocates expressed little interest in establishing a freestanding clinic independent of Planned Parenthood. For several years the local newspapers claimed that family planning services in Daleton were inferior to those of other communities. Editorials derided the presence of Catholic priests on the United Way Executive Board. Other news articles depicted the troubles at Planned Parenthood as a reflection of a liberal community held at bay by several priests attempting to impose Church doctrine on United Way policy. Ironically, the absence of support for a freestanding clinic in the community was less the result of religious forces than of professional expectations that physicians had about the role of family planning in medical work. These expectations were first developed during residency.

The four years of specialty training were salaried. A residency in obstetrics and gynecology marked the beginning of intensive clinical training in medicine and surgery. In addition to working with attendings (all of whom were physicians in private practice) and their patients, residents seeking clinical experience were encouraged to see patients who used the services of Planned Parenthood. The physician received an honorarium (four dollars) from Planned Parenthood for each patient seen. An obvious contrast existed between the fee-for-service charge of the private practitioner and the salary and symbolic remunerations of the resident physician. As the physician moved from residency to private practice, contact with this population of patients was maintained more symbolically than clinically.

Of the ten physicians who had done part or all of their residencies at Daleton Hospital, only three, all Catholic, had had no affiliation with the local Planned Parenthood clinic. Once in private practice, three who had worked at Planned Parenthood continued to serve on the clinic's Executive Board or on the Medical Advisory Committee, which monitored those residents who were clinically responsible for this service. The other physicians in private practice were grateful for the experience gained during their residencies, but as soon as their practices became busy they ended their clinical affiliations with Planned Parenthood. One referred to himself as an "advisory figurehead" who attended two Planned Parenthood board meetings a year.

Physician commitment to family planning as a public health and social service was determined by training requirements at different points along the way toward specialization in obstetrics and gynecology. Soon after the completion of residency, obstetrician/gynecologists at Daleton Hospital were put on a probation known as board eligible. Probation lasted until board certification was awarded by the American Board of Obstetrics and Gynecology. Since the board was incorporated in 1930, many hospitals have required that physicians claiming a specialty status become board certified within a stipulated amount of time following postdoctoral or residency training (see Wechsler, 1976:41).

Each specialty board (for example, the American Board of Ophthalmology, American Board of Dermatology, and American Board of Pediatrics) has established its own set of requirements specifying when a physician is permitted to apply for board certification examinations. The American Board of Obstetrics and Gynecology has required that graduates of residency programs in obstetrics and gynecology apply to take these examinations within three years after residency. Until passing the board examinations (or for three years, whichever comes first), the physician is normally given the same hospital privileges as those who are board certified. At Daleton Hospital, if a physician failed to take or pass the examinations, he could be asked to resign from the hospital staff.

David Mechanic has written that board certification "has no actual legal status" but "often brings higher salaries and higher payment under various public and private insurance programs" (1979:179). Staff policy at Daleton Hospital dictated that obstetrician/gynecologists be board certified. This policy guaranteed that the physician's competence met with the highest approval within his specialty. In recent years, the American Board of Obstetrics and Gynecology has been "authorized to qualify and examine candidates for a 'certificate of special competence' " in one of three specialty divisions within obstetrics and gynecology—gynecologic oncology, maternal and fetal medicine, and reproductive endocrinology (Wechsler, 1976:41). In order to receive this special certification, the physician must practice at least five years in one of these three subspecialties.

Board certification and certificates of special competence represent the specialty's and the hospital's recognition of physician achievement and medical-technical expertise. The need to devote time to these formal requirements discouraged obstetrician/gynecologists from routinely participating in family planning clinics as they trained further within their specializations. The American Board of Obstetrics and Gynecology did not require (and still does not require) participation in family planning clinics as part of a physician's professional certification. Work in such clinics was acknowledged by the board only in terms of the clinical experience acquired there.

As one of its eleven requirements for certification, the board asked that the physician "keep a record of the number and type of obstetric and gynecologic procedures performed during his residency, so that he can demonstrate the adequacy of his operative experience."[3] Routine physical examinations and contraceptive counseling were not considered sufficient evidence of clinical competence, and the performance of first-trimester abortions had a relatively low priority for doctors intent upon improving operative technique. Each doctor who had worked as a resident at the local Planned Parenthood facility discontinued the clinical affiliation in favor of seeing patients exclusively in private practice. For each, the acquisition of clinical experience was finally more important than the commitment to family planning as a social service.

All physicians indicated their willingness to counsel patients on family planning, but on terms that were not always the same as those of the local Planned Parenthood program. Several Catholic doctors took exception to the aims of Planned Parenthood, but not to the principle of family planning. Older practitioners had less and less to do with patients seeking birth control information or services. In addition to specialty and hospital requirements, both the personal convictions and the stage of career of physicians appeared to influence their lack of participation in a universally accepted program of family planning.

Religious Affiliation and Medical Practice

Obstetrician/gynecologists in Daleton were predominately Protestant (54% vs. 27% Catholic and 19% Jewish). Most of the Catholic physicians were based at St. Timothy. Jewish physicians, except the youngest one, who was in a group at Daleton Hospital, practiced alone and were on staff at Central or St. Timothy. They had worked in Daleton on average for more than twenty-five years. The fact that only one Jewish obstetrician/gynecologist had succeeded to the staff of the most prestigious hospital in the community revealed a legacy of discrimination that until recently had been clearly expressed in the pattern of hospital affiliations of most Jewish practitioners in all medical specialties in the community. A similar pattern was evident among Catholic doctors (see table 3.1).

St. Timothy formally prohibited its medical staff from performing

Table 3.1 | Religious and Hospital Affiliations of Obstetrician/
Gynecologists in Daleton

	Protestant	Catholic	Jewish
Daleton Hospital (N = 15)	11 (73%)	3 (20%)	1 (7%)
Central Hospital (N = 5)	3 (60%)	0 (0%)	2 (40%)
St. Timothy Hospital (N = 6)	0 (0%)	4 (67%)	2 (33%)

elective abortions and sexual sterilizations. The other two hospitals
had not promulgated such restrictions; administrators and physicians
at these institutions expected only that a doctor be medically and
technically competent in performing them. As long as these procedures were accepted in the law, professional standards formed the
basis for hospital policy at Daleton and Central.

Daleton's Protestant and Jewish obstetrician/gynecologists supported in principle a patient's right to choose any birth control option.
They did not have religious convictions against performing abortions.
For example, hospital policy at St. Timothy did not permit the two
Jewish practitioners on staff there to perform abortions or sterilizations despite the fact that these doctors regarded the procedures
as legitimate components of family planning. In their private practices,
the doctors were able to ignore hospital mandates about how to
practice medicine. Both had worked out a compromise of sorts by
joining the courtesy staff at Central, which allowed them to use the
operating facilities during weekday afternoons. They performed
elective first-trimester abortions and contraceptive sterilizations at
Central.

The Catholic group practice at St. Timothy (group five [see fig.
3.1]) maintained no affiliation with the local Planned Parenthood
facility. On rare occasions the agency made referrals to the group if
patients requested a Catholic physician. Both physicians in the group
prescribed the contraceptive pill to married patients, but not, as one
remarked, to "a sixteen-year-old kid coming in for pills." They justified
prescribing the pill to a married woman when, for example, there
were indications that her health might suffer if she were to become

pregnant too soon after delivering a child. One physician admitted that prescribing the pill was sometimes a convenient way to solve "several problems." Counseling in birth control by group five consisted of instruction in the rhythm method and the more sophisticated natural family planning method. The latter method is identical with the traditional rhythm method, except that it uses more elaborate means (including the taking of temperature) to determine precisely when ovulation is occurring.

A solo Catholic practitioner on staff at St. Timothy also prescribed the pill "on a limited basis." He would not fit diaphragms but favored their use rather than the IUD, which he called an abortifacient. With help from his nurses, he counseled exclusively in the rhythm method. His unwillingness to prescribe other methods set him apart from most of his fellow doctors, who endorsed all legal forms of birth control but expressed more enthusiasm for some than for others.

For most Catholic doctors, the conflict between professional competence and religious belief was profound. Given the availability in the community of other forms of birth control of which they did not approve, the Catholic physicians on staff at St. Timothy found themselves professionally isolated from their colleagues at other hospitals. Several physicians on staff at Daleton Hospital disparaged the idea that one could be a devout Catholic and a competent obstetrician/gynecologist.

The most serious charge made against Daleton's Catholic doctors came in reports that patients were not offered complete information about birth control options. One doctor spoke strongly against his Catholic colleagues on the matter of abortion referral: "I get absolutely no joy whatsoever doing any abortion, but we have a duty to an individual. The Catholic physician is aborting the Hippocratic Oath more than I am in not giving a woman the choice."

As will be further discussed in the next chapter, Daleton physicians could hardly be described as consistent in their use of referrals for abortion. The Catholic practitioner's dilemma was not unlike that of any doctor who did not offer abortion or other forms of birth control as a regular part of his medical practice. The intensity of criticism against the Catholics in particular signaled deeper rifts among physicians about the putative goals of family planning. For those who defended the entire spectrum of birth control methods,

Catholic intransigence was tantamount to professional incompetence. Viewed from the Catholic practitioner's side, the integrity of one's professional life was defined by convictions that transcended the changing nature of birth control technology and the changing character of professional responsibility.

Catholic physicians used another strategy for confronting the disparities among personal conviction, professional competence, and hospital policy. Two Catholic doctors practicing in active groups at Daleton Hospital had chosen to specialize in urology. Because they belonged to groups with large practices, they often saw patients referred specially to them by their partners. Such patients were unlikely to make demands on them for either birth control counseling or services. Protected by their private specialties, these doctors could lament the fact that abortion and sterilization were now widely accepted in the practice of medicine, but they tolerated their more liberal partners' work in these procedures.

The Catholic obstetrician/gynecologist typified one way in which personal conviction determined professional responsibility. For others, conviction was mediated by different experiences that were no less influential in determining how they viewed their professional responsibilities to patients and family planning.

Dr. Gardner's Generation

Older physicians (those who were born before 1931 or who were graduated from medical school before 1955) had acquired clinical experience with Planned Parenthood in Daleton under far different circumstances than their younger colleagues (see table 3.2). They also were more likely to be in solo practice. Dr. Gardner, for example,

Table 3.2 | Age Distribution of Obstetrician/Gynecologists in Daleton (N = 26)

Born		Graduated	
1911–20	5 (19%)	1935–45	6 (23%)
1921–30	7 (27%)	1946–55	5 (19%)
1931–40	7 (27%)	1956–65	6 (23%)
1941–50	7 (27%)	1966–75	9 (35%)

had begun in solo practice and then started what was now the oldest group practice in the community. When he began his practice in Daleton during the late 1930s, married couples were being encouraged to practice "family planning" under the guidance of trained specialists. Margaret Sanger, a leader of birth control reform in the United States, wrote in her often republished marriage manual, *Happiness in Marriage,* that "the safest and most hygienic methods [of birth control] cannot be used by the unmarried girl" (1939:210).[4] Sanger's warning reflected and strengthened professional and public expectations about who should use birth control.

The work that Dr. Gardner and colleagues of his generation did for Planned Parenthood in the early days of their medical careers was hardly controversial. For example, one of them counseled patients with infertility problems; another performed routine gynecological examinations. The propriety of sexual mores concealed a folklore of exceptions about who used birth control and what kinds of birth control were available. Two doctors practicing in Daleton for more than twenty years mentioned a local nurse who was known to have performed abortions before 1973.[5]

For the older practitioners in Daleton, family planning was the least important component of their practices. Dr. Gardner remarked that he was not well trained in performing abortions or in the insertion of the IUD, but he carefully studied the literature on the uses of estrogen during menopause. His patient load had declined in recent years. By working in a group practice he could have seen more patients. Instead, he allowed his practice to dwindle, first by referring all obstetrical cases to his partners and then by refusing to take on any new gynecological cases. Another older member of Dr. Gardner's group had found that one way to supplement his patient load was to perform abortions and sexual sterilizations on request. He relied on his younger colleagues for referrals.

Dr. Tobin, a solo practitioner in her mid-sixties and the only female physician practicing obstetrics and gynecology in Daleton, spoke highly of her long association with Planned Parenthood. For more than thirty years she had advocated the use of diaphragms and condoms. She remarked with indignation that "men are very egotistical about their sexuality and many husbands won't use condoms." Furthermore,

If it were up to me, there would only be diaphragms. I don't think to this day that the fitting of them is taught in medical school. I've never been on the bandwagon for the pill or IUD. The pill is very convenient, but I don't like to tamper with hormones. I don't approve of the IUD at all. I don't have it in my office. There is definitely a hazard. I've removed many IUDs because of chronic infection.

Dr. Tobin observed that in her clinical experience many women sought the services of Planned Parenthood only after one or more abortions. Her generation of medical practitioners had not been initially trained in either abortion techniques or the use of such birth control technologies as the IUD and the oral contraceptive.

In assessing the use of such technologies, Dr. Tobin emphasized three different problems: male reluctance to use birth control, the lack of training of medical students in family planning, and the risks associated with the pill and IUD. Unlike her Catholic colleagues, who were determined to combine religious conviction with professional practice, Dr. Tobin, who was Jewish, was guided by beliefs about individual responsibility and harm. Birth control was less a technical means to desired ends than a morally complex set of responsibilities that physicians and patients had to confront. Her perspective is further illuminated by disputes among other physicians about how best to fulfill these responsibilities in the face of the demands of medical practice.

Family Planning in Two Group Practices

Dr. Ingram of group four had been a partner in group one for ten years until the mid-1970s, when he decided to open his own group practice with Dr. Jones, who had only recently joined group one. By then, Dr. Ingram had established a large enough practice to make the move economically feasible. He also expressed reservations about the group one approach to family planning. From the beginning, his ideological falling out with Dr. Simpson, the head of group one, was intensified by personal conflicts between them.

Dr. Ingram was satisfied that Dr. Simpson offered the necessary medical services for modern family planning (for example, in-office abortions and contraceptive sterilizations), but he accused him of not giving the counseling that Dr. Ingram believed had to go along with these services: "Seeing a patient with a problem pregnancy and counseling her for three minutes [before agreeing to perform an abortion] may not be enough, considering the woman may have been struggling with related problems [e.g., sexual and emotional problems] for the last ten years." Referring patients to the clinics outside Daleton was, no doubt, a strategic way of avoiding the "related problems." Dr. Ingram distinguished between the physician's responsibility to enable patients to achieve control over their reproduction and the responsibility to encourage a particular kind of control, preferably one that would reduce the resort to abortion.

Dr. Ingram argued that a physician who did not offer counseling might accept abortion and sterilization as *whole* solutions to problems that he hoped could be resolved in other ways: "When you look at abortion or sterilization, you can see it in two ways I guess. One sees it as a help, to improve society. Or one sees the necessity to keep the numbers of dirty, poor people down. I'm not Jewish, I'm not a historian, but not only Jews need to worry about the mentality that allows this sort of thing to happen." If birth control was to be a social improvement and not a social necessity, he believed, counseling would have to assume a prominent place in the physician's practice. The physician would be expected to treat each physician-patient interaction as personally, if not clinically, unique. Abortion and sterilization, he argued, should be made available, but their abuses could be diminished only through the mutual understanding and trust of physician and patient: "In my relationship to somebody regarding family planning, a whole individual's life is reflected. It reflects the presence or absence of the life of another individual. It gets you into the very subjective area of sexuality." Like Dr. Tobin, Dr. Ingram described the morally complex reality of family planning that physicians could choose or not choose to confront. Unlike his Catholic colleagues, his ambivalence arose over how birth control services were given, not over whether they should be given. He remained uncertain about how best to encourage patients to rely more on themselves and less on doctors for their control of conception.

In his report of a conversation with a former chief resident, Dr. Ingram offered various reasons for the failure in family planning pedagogy:

> We were talking about a woman we had sterilized, with psychiatric problems, who had never had children but who believed she was a potential child abuser. Then we got into a discussion about repeaters [those who

have more than one abortion]. The resident said he would never do a second abortion on the same woman because of her failure to use contraception. I think you have to look at the problem of repeaters in a different way.

First, I ask myself how much is this my fault. I have no business being angry with her. Next, I think there is something wrong with the medical system, and the counseling is not effective enough. And is it good to proceed with a second unplanned pregnancy when the first unplanned one was terminated?

Resort to abortion, in contrast to the use of other forms of birth control, was viewed as a failure (however inevitable) in family planning. The sources of this failure, as he described them, were more political than moral. He blamed himself, the "medical system," and ineffective counseling but refused to moralize about a patient's behavior. Nevertheless, to preserve the moral implications of that failure without having to advocate the outlawing of abortion, he stressed the importance of finding ways to reduce the need for the procedure.

Dr. Ingram, and most of his colleagues, believed that reproduction could be controlled in better and worse ways. But the meanings of better and worse were complicated by the different weights given to the variables of safety and convenience and to the notions of individual and social responsibility. Sexual sterilization (of females and males) was highly regarded as a safe and efficient method of birth control. They all qualified their enthusiasm for this procedure for women who were under thirty or who had no children. Mechanical methods (for example, diaphragms and condoms), they noted, could be used ineffectively but were safer for many users than the IUD or the pill. What was sacrificed in convenience was made up for in the reduction of risk to health. Physicians mentioned that the pill was the most often requested method of contraception among their patients.

Dr. Ingram was convinced that most people would not accept or follow the rhythm method. He mentioned a friend who had once contemplated becoming a priest and who practiced the "scientific" rhythm method with his wife: "Taking smears of cervical mucus and taking temperatures requires too much manipulation and fussiness. Experience shows that large numbers of people don't have the motivation for that kind of messing around." Dr. Ingram's judgment about patient motivation was an important factor in his estimation of what kinds of birth control were likely to be used successfully. Many Daleton physicians were especially pessimistic about the likelihood that males would take responsibility for birth control. On the basis of what "experience shows," Dr. Ingram rejected the idea that large numbers of people could be motivated to adopt a less medically involved control of conception. Having blamed himself, the medical system, and poor counseling for the present state of family planning, he acknowledged the limits of pedagogy as well as a seemingly uncontrollable feature of human nature, in this case psychologized as motivation.

Most of Dr. Ingram's colleagues were not as hard on themselves or their profession. One recalled three instances within the year when a patient had requested a second abortion after he had performed one for her. He described these patients as having "poor images" of themselves: "She can't remember to take the pill from day to day. Everything turns to shit for them." Other doctors worried more about the potential consequences of overpopulation. Although many had prescribed and continued to offer the IUD, they believed it was better suited for nations with rapid population growth than for more or less stable societies. In the United States, two groups, the young and the poor, were mentioned most often as the least able to practice birth control without the aid of such medical technologies as the IUD.

An older practitioner on staff at Daleton Hospital contended that family planning services were reaching the wrong people: "A high percentage of people on welfare are going to have lots of grandchildren. This thing is going to mushroom and we are going to lose the backbone which makes the U.S. a world leader." Other ob/gyns in Daleton defended family planning on economic grounds. In their support for federal funding for abortion, for example, they did not emphasize their right to perform the procedure (or a patient's right to receive it) but rather the national need to make it available:

> Those [young and poor] are the ones that need it most. There are so many damn welfare programs. It's like spitting in the ocean. Here is a positive program—the kids live in an environment that doesn't offer much hope. I don't think we are going to lose very many Napoleons or Beethovens doing this. . . . The population problem is not caused by the off-

spring of young engineers or doctors—the fewer of these, the fewer there
will be to support those who don't limit their offspring. If we don't do
something about it, we will populate ourselves off the earth. That's suicide,
slow suicide. That's one solution.

Such views were generously offered, and they reflected the popular
liberal argument that "environment" is a major determinant of a person's life chances. The "positive program" of birth control also evoked
eugenic sentiments. Doctors advocated it as a solution to "so many
damn welfare programs" and to "slow suicide." It was both a social
improvement and a social necessity.

Among all the obstetrician/gynecologists in Daleton, Dr. Simpson
was the strongest and most articulate supporter of the work of
Planned Parenthood in the community. He was director of the residency program in obstetrics and gynecology at Daleton Hospital
and was well known among his colleagues for his work in sexual
sterilization and abortion. He was working on a surgical improvement
in tubal ligations that he hoped would eventually make this form of
sterilization surgically reversible. His technical modifications of the
laparoscope (an instrument for diagnostic surgery) had earned him
recognition outside the community. He had published several papers
on the outcomes of numerous laparoscopic sterilizations performed
at Daleton Hospital.

Dr. Simpson proudly claimed that he often prescribed contraceptives and performed abortions for patients who in other circumstances
used the services of the Catholic group practice based at St. Timothy:
"My name is sort of mud with the Catholics in town, with Catholic
priests. I've never been placarded, though they did once bring out
all these kids from the Catholic schools to march around the front
of the hospital." Many of the physicians on staff at Daleton Hospital
recalled this "parade," but none was aware of any comparable incident
in which public protests were directed against the performing of
abortions there.

After the legalization of abortion in 1973, Dr. Simpson used a
procedure known as menstrual extraction or aspiration, a technique
of inducing menstruation artificially in a patient who suspects that
she is pregnant. He was thus able to offer another means of birth
control to those who were ambivalent about abortion. Another physician in the community referred to menstrual aspiration as a "D &

C [dilation and curettage] by any other name."[6] Dr. Simpson eventually abandoned the procedure as a birth control method when he found that medical complications sometimes occurred: "Doing a first-trimester abortion is a much simpler and easier procedure. It's much easier to prove pregnancy, then abort; otherwise in MA [menstrual aspiration] you have to keep rechecking afterwards to make sure you got everything out. She [the patient] must be followed with MA, but abortion is once and done with one follow-up." Dr. Ingram agreed with his former partner that menstrual extraction was unnecessarily invasive surgery when used specifically for suspected pregnancy, and he thought that the women's movement had done "people a disservice in advocating menstrual extraction as a routine form of birth control" (see also Hern, 1984:120–122).

Dr. Simpson's voice boomed with assurance when he offered his opinions about birth control and family planning:

> Men don't like to use condoms. It's like washing your feet with socks on. Men are not as reliable. They don't go for routine annual physicals. . . . A prick has no conscience. Unless a man has mature control over his sexuality, forget it! . . . No man owns his wife's tubes. . . . You should think of abortion like a linebacker in football. . . . The young pregnant girl needs a mother, she doesn't need to be a mother. We need ZPG [zero population growth], we are overpopulated. Just travel around. There are too goddamn many people in the world. The family with four and five children is leaving our American heritage. In India they say, "Don't give us fifty million dollars, give us birth control!" I'm told by sociologists that India is not going to survive. There are 10,000 starving a day I think.

His reaction to the question of how he would deal with overpopulation was equally candid but hardly serious:

> My wife [also a physician] and I traveled across America and drove through North Dakota and looked at all the space. But on the Eastern seaboard, the urban areas, they are overpopulated. I swear I'm going to do more laparoscopies [sexual sterilizations] whenever I'm in line having to wait to use the restroom in a restaurant or waiting in traffic.

Dr. Ingram took personal offense at Dr. Simpson's sense of humor more than at his views about birth control and family planning. In fact, the two doctors did not disagree in principle about their professional responsibilities to offer patients the complete spectrum of birth control options. Their dispute over counseling patients about these options (particularly abortion) reflected differences in both the style and the substance of their medical practices.

Dr. Simpson said that he performed abortions most frequently for teenagers: "I've had one who I've done four abortions for, and she is 24 years old. I've had a 12-year-old who has had three—they get a hell of a lecture from me and they're all counseled. I do it [the abortion] reluctantly." Because he also considered the resort to abortion as a failure in family planning, Dr. Simpson insisted that patients receive contraceptive counseling. He himself did not often give this counseling. Instead, patients were referred to one of the nurses in the group who specialized in this work. He commented: "Margaret does all the counseling. As a woman, a married woman and a mother, patients identify better with her." Dr. Ingram, on the other hand, claimed that he and his partner always provided such counseling themselves. But they provided much less of it. Dr. Simpson devoted at least 30 percent of his time to performing sterilizations and abortions (that is, nonobstetrical family planning), 30 percent to obstetrical cases, and 40 percent to routine gynecological treatments and surgeries. Dr. Ingram gave at least half his time to obstetrical cases and to treatments for infertility (that is, obstetrical family planning), 10 percent to birth control counseling, and 40 percent to routine gynecological cases other than birth prevention.

Dr. Ingram's split from group one was ironic for several reasons. He argued that he began his own group because he objected to his former group's approach to nonobstetrical family planning in particular. Yet, in his new group practice, neither he nor his partner had given much thought to devising means to improve what he considered wrong with that approach. He confirmed this in remarks about his wife's work in Planned Parenthood: "My wife's involvement has been very, very extensive—hours and hours and hours of involvement on the national and state level, and the local level and so on. I think it's affected me more in my personal life than it has in my professional practice because of her involvement and the pressures. It hasn't changed my day-to-day work one iota." The demands of his practice were already considerable. Even though he was licensed by the state to perform in-office abortions (only Dr. Simpson's group had a similar license), he believed he could not "put many more hours in this office and maintain any kind of life." Nonobstetrical family planning was more a political calling for his wife than a medical one for him.

Routine obstetrical and gynecological work had also reduced the time that Dr. Ingram could allot to infertility cases. He placed an upper limit on the number of patients he thought he could serve in gynecology, but he claimed that obstetrical cases were never turned away:

> We don't have a mechanism yet by which we can limit or have limited the number of OB patients. We really don't know how to do that. It's done. I have a patient who wanted to stay here, deliver, rather than go out to Michigan. Her husband is out at Ann Arbor, the university town. You have doctors falling all over each other. She said, "My God! I've called several people and they're not taking any new patients." Well, at that particular point they have all the patients they were going to register for that particular month. And they said, "No." We haven't come to that yet! How do you have your thirty people listed by the 20th of July or on the 23rd of July and somebody who has been delivered twice before or whatever, and you say "no" to them?

Obstetrical family planning (including work in infertility) continued to be more important in Dr. Ingram's practice of medicine than non-obstetrical family planning. His thoughtful, often ambivalent, remarks about the aims of family planning were finally reflected in how he chose to organize his medical practice.

By keeping his group practice relatively small, Dr. Ingram hoped that he could serve his patients better. He also believed that larger groups were expected to be more active in their provision of non-obstetrical family planning services, especially abortion and sterili-zation. Despite his wife's efforts on behalf of Planned Parenthood, he continued to practice medicine impervious to outside pressures. When asked about new treatments for infertility, such as in vitro fertilization, he observed:

> Yes, I have some people who will be candidates for referral. No doubt about it. It's a different point about what do I think about the whole topic. I have a little trouble about my own attitude about this, because on one level I said to myself a few times, "Jesus! Given where we are in this world now, is this an appropriate investment in dollars, or barrels of oil, or whatever the hell you're going to pay for it in? Is it really?" That

produces a little bit of a question that I raised to myself, it produces a little bit of a dilemma, because indeed I feel that I have rather strong obligations to those people who come to me expecting and hoping that I have some measure of expertise in helping them to achieve pregnancy.

A sense of professional responsibility superseded political and economic assessments of the best ways to practice medicine. The technical challenges of infertility were no doubt as attractive to Dr. Ingram as the technical challenges of laparoscopy were to Dr. Simpson. Their dispute revealed not only personal and ideological differences in their approaches to obstetrics and gynecology but also the social conditions of private practice that enabled them to pursue those approaches without interference (see Tschetter, 1978).

Obstetrician/gynecologists have assumed responsibility for family planning in its most technologically sophisticated forms. From treatments for infertility to fetal monitoring (that is, obstetrical family planning) and from prescription of the pill to the performance of abortion and sterilization (that is, nonobstetrical family planning), they have acted with differing convictions about the best ways to practice in this specialty. Daleton physicians' choices about how to practice were guided by factors other than religious belief, stage of career, and specialization within obstetrics and gynecology. Examining their attitudes and practices regarding abortion will allow us to see more clearly the separation of birthing from birth controlling.

4
The First-Trimester Abortion: Standard Procedures

Ten of the twenty-six obstetrician/gynecologists (38.5%) in Daleton said they were willing to perform abortions on request, but on terms that were neither universal nor consistent. Ten others (38.5%) had performed abortions at one time or another but, for reasons to be explored here, had stopped doing so. The remaining six (23%), all Catholics, indicated that they had never performed an elective abortion.[1] Of those physicians who accepted or had at one time accepted requests for elective abortion (77%), only two were now willing to perform the procedure after the first trimester of pregnancy. In this chapter, I will describe how physicians negotiated requests for first-trimester abortions.

Physicians' rationales for accepting or refusing requests for abortion were expressed in the contexts of their solo or group practices, where the use of referrals was common. Despite the fact that most doctors considered a first-trimester abortion to be a technically simple and standard procedure, some cited concern for their professional identity in the larger community as an important reason for referring patients elsewhere. Private practices and professional reputations were interrelated, and physicians had little reason to challenge how abortions were made available. In addition to the social contexts of private practice, the training experiences of physicians influenced how they eventually handled requests for abortion. In particular, several younger practitioners who were trained outside Daleton decided no longer to perform elective abortions. Their conscientious objections, though not formally religious in origin, exemplified a conflict of convictions that lay at the heart of their medical view of abortion.

Referrals and Private Practice

Each year, 90 percent of all abortions in the United States are performed during the first trimester of pregnancy. The remaining 10 percent are performed during the second trimester—that is, between the twelfth and twenty-fourth weeks of pregnancy (see Centers for Disease Control, 1980, 1983, and National Abortion Rights Action League, 1978:12).

Methods used to perform abortions have evolved rapidly since the early 1970s. An abortion in the first trimester is usually performed between the seventh and tenth weeks of pregnancy. The most frequently used method prior to 1973 was dilation and curettage (D & C). This requires dilating the cervix in order to enter the uterus with a sharp metal curette. The "products of conception" are then scraped carefully from the interior lining of the uterus.[2] Since the early 1970s, vacuum aspiration of the uterus has gained wider recognition and is now the preferred method of termination, especially in the first trimester. More recently it has been modified and is now used in the second trimester up to eighteen to twenty weeks (Bolognese and Corson, 1975).

The vacuum aspirator, or suction machine, technique utilizes a curette-like tube, or cannula. Cervical dilation is necessary when a rigid cannula is used, but with a more flexible tube dilation is unnecessary if the pregnancy is less than ten weeks. The risks associated with first-trimester abortion—for example, perforation of the uterus, incomplete evacuation of the uterus, and sepsis (infection)—have been significantly reduced. With the flexible cannula and the vacuum aspirator, discomfort to the patient has also been lessened, except for cramping in the uterus during aspiration. Dilation of the cervix may occasionally be necessary if the physician determines that the pregnancy is further along than was originally believed. In such cases, the risk of damaging the cervix is increased.

Improvements in surgical instrumentation and technique have reduced the risk and discomfort to patients and made the first-trimester abortion a relatively safe operation, easily performed on an outpatient basis. Two group practices (groups one and four) had obtained state licenses to perform first-trimester abortions in their offices. In fact only group one performed them there; group four referred elective requests elsewhere. (One member said that having the license kept the group "professionally up to date.") Other physicians in the community admitted patients to Daleton or Central Hospital or referred them to clinics in nearby cities. On rare occasions, a doctor would refer a patient to another colleague in the community for a first-trimester abortion (see fig. 4.1).

In *Passage Through Abortion: The Personal and Social Reality of Women's Experiences,* Mary K. Zimmerman described two "routes" that a woman could typically take in order to obtain an abortion: the "traditional medicine route" and the "specialized clinic alternative." In the first case, "a woman suspects that she is pregnant and contacts her physician; the physician confirms the pregnancy and either arranges to perform an abortion in a local hospital or refers the woman to another physician who will." In the second case, "the woman contacts the public health department's family-planning clinic to have her pregnancy confirmed." She is then referred to a freestanding clinic that is, as Zimmerman described it, "devoted primarily to performing abortions" (1977:33–34).

Daleton group and solo practitioners had initiated various strategies to respond to requests for elective abortions. In order to travel successfully along the traditional medicine route described by Zimmerman, a patient had to establish contact with a physician in either of these types of medical practice. Direct contact with a private physician was not always easily accomplished. For example, when group two at Daleton Hospital first formed, the three partners agreed to perform elective first-trimester abortions. More recently they had decided to have the appointments secretary refer the few requests for abortions that came over the telephone to abortion clinics in nearby cities. The doctors, once they had confirmed pregnancy, referred regular patients requesting abortion to these same clinics.

The two members of group six at Central Hospital maintained a similar policy toward telephone requests and patient referral. The

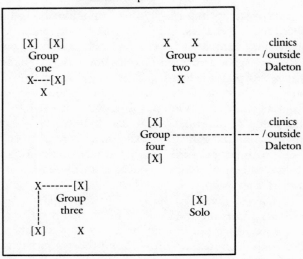

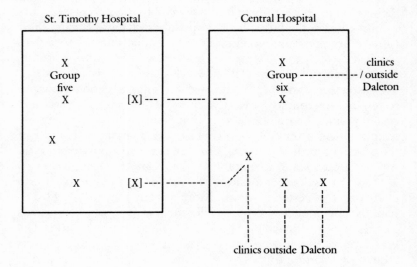

Figure 4.1 Patterns of Abortion Referral in Daleton. [X]-performed elective abortions.

appointments secretary occupied a strategic position in redirecting patients to other service providers. Those patients who were already known to the physicians received a different kind of attention than did patients who called for the first time requesting an abortion. Dr. Evans of group six stated:

> Well, you know, there's a lot of inconsistencies. I say I'm opposed to it and I tell my people where to go to get them. I don't really even do that very much. My instruction to my office staff is that if they want an abortion to tell them that we just don't deal in that at all. And they do have a few phone numbers that they can give to these people. But if I get one back here and I get involved in it, I'll counsel them and sort of help them to make their decision.

The physician's motivation to aid a patient in search of an abortion was rarely consistent, especially when a group had decided to refer elective abortion requests elsewhere. These inconsistencies remained unnoticed if one had contact only with the appointments secretary. The organization of private practice permitted doctors to handle a standard, legal, and relatively safe procedure on their own less standard but perfectly legal terms. By offering information about referrals, they also believed that they were fulfilling their medical obligations to patients.

Several group practices in Daleton contained members who were willing to perform abortions on request. In each of these groups, explicit understandings existed among colleagues about who would and who would not perform them. The appointments secretary often referred patients directly to one of the physicians in the group who would. Those who would not thereby avoided negotiating such requests. In one group, a recently arrived member was assigned offices one flight up from those of his new partners. At first sight, the physical separation could be explained by the need for more space, but it was also symbolic: the new member worked exclusively with obstetrical patients, while his partners one floor below did primarily gynecological work, including abortions and nonobstetrical family planning.

Solo practitioners unwilling to perform elective abortions used referrals in ways similar to those used by the group doctors. Several assumed that most abortions in the community were performed by their younger colleagues. It is important to remember that many of these doctors had been in practice in Daleton for more than twenty years. A practitioner in his late fifties remarked, "We were always admonished against doing abortions in medical school. I don't want to be known as an abortionist." Despite changes in the law, the stricture persisted. Being able to make legal referrals gave him a great sense of relief, and he was no longer haunted by the requests made of him when abortion was illegal. A referral represented a compromise between his medical education and ambivalent feelings about wanting to help in such situations. For years he could do little other than recommend adoption. At one point he bitterly remarked, "I've always wondered about what would happen to a forty-five-year-old right-to-lifer if she became pregnant." He felt professionally obligated to mention all legal alternatives even though he was personally reluctant to participate directly in making all of them available.

The last chapter mentioned two solo practitioners who were on staff at St. Timothy but performed elective abortions and sterilizations at Central. One of them was "sincerely happy if they go somewhere else." He said several times that he "really didn't have that many abortions to do" and that he regularly referred patients requesting them to the clinics outside Daleton. The other, Dr. Roth, often accepted abortion referrals from a colleague, Dr. Adams, who was on staff at Central.

Dr. Adams also served on the faculties of two teaching hospitals and maintained a small private practice in a community about two hours north of Daleton. He was licensed to practice medicine in four states: "My practice consists in the vast majority of referrals. I'm a doctor's doctor. I do the surgery which the others would just as soon not do." For a time, such surgery included abortions. Following the liberalization of abortion laws, he actively performed the procedure for anyone requesting it, but in recent years he had grown disaffected. He now referred requests to Dr. Roth because he believed that performing abortions had become "dirty work"[3]: "The state medical school hospital [where he taught] had a clinic for first-trimester abortions, but it has been closed down for over a year because they were getting ripped off a great deal." More and more patients requesting abortions, he claimed, were not paying for them. He described them as "California types who were in town one week and gone for good the next."

Dr. Adams referred patients "down" to Dr. Roth in the same way that he believed other physicians referred patients "up" to him. Dr. Roth was not necessarily less competent at performing abortions than his colleagues, but Dr. Adams no longer viewed them as challenging or innovative, and, in any case, he had changed his opinion of many patients requesting them. Other physicians gave a more positive rationale for referring patients to the clinics: they claimed that the clinics were better equipped technically and psychologically for abortion. In Daleton, abortion referral was an expression of deference and of avoidance, as all referrals are. To avoid abortion meant also to avoid controversy—no other surgery has been associated so much with court litigation, human rights, and medical morality. Referral was the privilege to say no without having to take a public stand on any of these matters.

Technical Standards and Professional Identity

Dr. Simpson of group one looked on abortion as an essential part of family planning. He estimated that he performed about a hundred of them in his office each year. Although he agreed that medical indications existed for abortion, he was most concerned about performing procedures safely and efficiently. He did not perform them after the first trimester. His reason was straightforward: terminations of pregnancy after twelve weeks were technically more complicated, and he could not perform them in his office. Until 1983, many states required physicians to perform abortions beyond the first trimester in hospitals.[4]

Having abandoned menstrual aspiration as a family planning method in the mid-1970s, Dr. Simpson remarked that its advantage over abortion for some patients did not outweigh the medical complications he had treated after the procedure. He preferred to perform first-trimester abortions between eight and ten weeks of pregnancy using the vacuum-aspiration method because he encountered the fewest complications operatively and postoperatively (see Centers for Disease Control, 1980, 1983). His acceptance of this procedure depended on its medically noncontroversial status.

Dr. Simpson accepted abortion as long as medical complications could be strictly limited. Another type of surgery could pose a greater risk than an elective first-trimester abortion, but in such a case, the risk was not inconsistent with good medical practice. In his mind, abortion was not intended to make a patient "well" again as was his expectation with some other medical treatments, such as surgery for a benign tumor. The risk associated with performing an abortion therefore had to be reduced as much as possible. He accepted those cases that posed the least risk to himself and the patient. Like all the other Daleton physicians who were willing to perform elective abortions in the first trimester, Dr. Simpson referred second-trimester abortion requests to Dr. Hill, whose reasons for accepting them are described in the next chapter.

Technical standards for first-trimester abortion not only were established by the physician's knowledge of the safest time and most efficient method for performing the procedure but also depended on what risks a patient was likely to face in undergoing it. One physician mentioned that he had read about an increase in cervical incompetence as a result of first-trimester abortions: "I mentioned to a woman just yesterday that she might have more difficulty conceiving and bearing a child after an abortion—I said it's a chance. You must be careful how to say this to a patient." By informing patients about the risks involved in undergoing a procedure, physicians spoke from personal experience, from their reading of the medical literature, and, just as often, on the basis of reports in the media. Physician-scientists have been increasingly called upon to clarify the risks associated with abortion, and predictably, scientific testimony has not persuaded either side in the larger political debate (compare Bondeson et al., 1983, and Hilgers et al., 1981; see also Maine, 1979, and Hogue et al., 1983).[5]

Daleton physicians differed about the scientific evidence regarding the harm caused by abortion. More important, they differed about the circumstances in which it was right and appropriate for them to perform one. No physician argued that the procedure was unsafe to life or health if performed under the best technical conditions. To this extent, avoiding abortion on medical-technical grounds was not the issue. Yet none of the obstetrician/gynecologists in Daleton, not even those who accepted elective requests, was fully consistent in his or her judgments about when to perform one.

With the improved health of women of reproductive age and the legalization of abortion, discussions about when the procedure was medically indicated became less prominent in the professional literature.[6] Yet the legacy of these discussions among physicians in medical practice continued. An "elective" abortion usurped the physician's traditional responsibility for determining what counted as medical treatment. Daleton physicians did not look upon pregnancy as life threatening precisely because they were better able than ever before to control its outcome. Medical control of the prevention of conception developed in the absence of legal access to abortion. The pill and sexual sterilization represent medically acceptable ways to prevent conception. Abortion, unlike the pill, requires that physicians take responsibility for birth control. Sexual sterilization offers a surgical way to prevent conception once and for all and thus eliminates the need for abortion as a form of birth control. Behind the public use of referrals, many physicians privately expressed widely varying rationales for their decision to perform or not to perform abortions.

Of those physicians who accepted elective requests for abortion, one argued that there were only "two logical directions to go in": either one believed that under no circumstance should a pregnancy be terminated, a position he described as "just plain stupid," or one believed that under any circumstance a woman should have the right to decide to end a pregnancy, which he found "abhorrent": "God's not talking to me, I'm not talking to the angels. I have a right to choose my point of when to do and when not to do an abortion, despite the fact that it is hypocritical, illogical. In my own moral frame, there are certain reasons, excuses, which do not justify my performing an abortion." He found "abhorrent" the idea of performing an abortion for parents who did not want a particular child because of its gender, as determined by amniocentesis during the second trimester of pregnancy. Another physician who regularly performed elective abortions insisted that he would "follow through on any request." Later in the same interview he said that he did not accept gender determination as a valid reason for ending a pregnancy and that, if ever asked for that reason, he would refer the patient elsewhere. The dilemma for him was moot, however, because he would not perform abortions beyond the first trimester.

Dr. Evans of group six was typical of several physicians who had once performed elective abortions but now required that medical indications exist before doing them:

The little biological body is not a human soul and it doesn't bother me taking a little biological life. I am opposed to destroying a living thing, I hate to shoot a bird or step on a bug or cut a beautiful plant, but I do. These things [abortions] are not done lightly. A lot of consideration and prayer is called for.

His attitude toward sexual behavior was more indicative of why he had changed his mind about elective abortion than was his speculation about the value of life or prayer. Like other physicians in the community, he believed that abortion was most problematic for teenagers:

> I would like to see abortions limited to cases where there is a serious threat to emotional and physical health, or rape and incest. There are too many people enjoying sex without paying attention to their acts. Babies are needed for adoption, although I do think there are very valid reasons for abortions sometimes. I just do not like the electives. . . . It is too god-damn easy for teenagers to screw. I have lectured in schools about the medical complications associated with adolescent intercourse. They don't like morality, but they sure like the facts.

He reacted strongly against the prospects for "do-it-yourself" abortion kits because "the public is not morally ready for them. It would be inviting people to be promiscuous."

Dr. Adams, who was several years older than Dr. Evans but had also done his residency during the late 1950s, said he abided by the criteria for therapeutic abortion developed from the Model Penal Code proposal of that time and later endorsed by the American College of Obstetricians and Gynecologists. Both doctors defended the right of physicians to perform elective abortions. The physician's privilege to decide when an abortion was indicated mattered more to them than any collective attempt to forge universal standards for all physicians. Having changed their professional views about the procedure, they once again appealed to criteria learned during residency. These older criteria became the ostensible basis upon which they accepted or refused requests for abortion.

Dr. Adams' change of mind was also influenced by judicial rulings that, in effect, discouraged physicians from performing abortions. In June 1977, the Supreme Court *(Beal v. Doe)* upheld state laws that prohibited state and local governments from subsidizing abortions "unless they were necessary to preserve the life or health of the person."[7] Daleton happened to be in one of the states that had passed a law requiring physicians to demonstrate the "therapeutic" necessity of a procedure in order to justify state reimbursement of the costs. Patients who received public welfare assistance were otherwise not eligible to have abortions paid for by the state.

In a letter responding to my inquiry about the new changes in the law, Dr. Adams wrote:

> Your "informant" has heard from many sources that the role of the illegal "abortionist" will expand as a result of this State, and many states, eliminating payment for "elective" pregnancy termination. Undoubtedly, the old dodge of "psychiatric indications" will resume increasing popularity, as elective terminations again become classified as "therapeutic" terminations.

The requirement of a signature on an affidavit attesting that a particular abortion was medically indicated meant that Dr. Adams was no longer guaranteed an income from performing elective abortions. He appeared to lower his opinion of patients who did not or could not pay for abortions at approximately the same time the state law was changed. His dissatisfaction with this change was to some extent taken out on those patients, who had not previously posed a financial burden to his medical practice. Above all, he objected to the idea of having to justify to the state or to patients his decision to agree or refuse to perform an abortion.[8]

Dr. Evans, on the other hand, stressed his professional identity and the reputation of his medical practice in the community when explaining why he no longer performed elective abortions. He and his younger partner had decided to take their obstetrical practice in a new direction. They were critical of the program at Daleton Hospital and the staff's attitude toward childbirth.

Under Dr. Evans' direction, group six and its nursing staff had instituted childbirth courses and birthing rooms at Central Hospital. The innovations were applauded in an article in the local newspaper:

> Dr. Evans brought the head and shoulders of baby Kaye into the world. Then, Mrs. Webster took baby Kaye's shoulders and brought the rest of baby Kaye's body out of hers and placed the infant on her stomach. No longer does the father have to pace back and forth in the waiting room. Now he can be an active participant, supplying much-needed moral support. The Websters, both teachers, wholeheartedly recommend that expectant parents take a course in childbirthing.

The doctors expected to train and license nurse-midwives and to open a separate birthing facility near Central. They described their role in the birthing rooms as that of advisers who were available in the event of emergency. In contrast to the "take charge" attitude typical of many obstetricians, these doctors hoped to create a new environment for obstetrical care. They did not oppose home births but offered their own approach as a convenient and safe alternative to regular hospital delivery.

Dr. Evans' decision to refer all but therapeutic abortions was finally formed by a combination of personal sentiments about the sexuality of teenagers, professional expectations from his residency about when abortion was indicated, and practical concerns about how his medical practice was publicly regarded:

> I hate doing them, but I do them every once in a while. But the real reason we try to avoid them is that I don't want to be known in the community as a local abortionist. I want to be known as a doctor who loves mommies and their babies. I don't care what is said, there is a stigma attached to doing abortions. There are political reasons not to earn the reputation as the local abortionist, I mean, to be known as the physician who will perform abortions whenever asked. My motivations are not selfish. We are working to bring to this community alternative ways for women to have their babies.

His efforts to educate expectant parents—and other physicians—about alternative approaches to childbirth would be threatened, he believed, by the perception that he was an abortionist.

In the last chapter, obstetrical family planning was contrasted to nonobstetrical family planning, thus suggesting a conflict about how Daleton physicians reconciled each type of work in their medical practices. The contrast between abortion work in particular and obstetrics revealed this conflict more clearly. The obstetrician is committed to protecting the mother and newborn as well as possible. The gynecologist who ends a pregnancy deliberately is committed to ensuring that the patient's life is protected while the fetus is removed. If a contradiction existed between the two types of work, it was resolved by referring elsewhere patients who requested abortions, by redefining the circumstances under which the procedure would be performed, or by establishing a medical practice limited ostensibly to either obstetrics or gynecology.[9] All these strategies were evident among physicians in Daleton. This is not to argue that they were unable to balance both types of work in their busy medical practices. Rather, by working in private practices, they were able to choose how that balance was achieved.[10]

Daleton physicians were reluctant to support the opening of a freestanding clinic in the community that would offer abortion services. Busy medical practices concealed one motive for their proceeding carefully in this regard. Despite the fact that several physicians could perform abortions discreetly in hospitals, the stigma of being labeled an abortionist hovered over them in the community. Dr. Ingram of group four, for example, performed elective abortions for patients he had known for a long period of time, but he referred other requests to clinics outside the community. He noted a connection between professional identity and the price of abortion: "In Daleton, the price of abortion is punitive. I think there is a price-fixing to avoid the abortionist stigma. You get patients coming to you who can afford it, and they want the whole thing to be discreet in the first place, whereas if you are known to do abortions, you would have them flocking to your door, and there isn't very much discreet about that." The abortionist stigma was in essence sociological; it arose not from doing abortions but from being *known* to do them. Keeping the price of abortion high, Dr. Ingram contended, reduced the probability of being stigmatized. Higher-priced services and referrals became public symbols of good reputation in the community.

The number of abortions performed in Daleton on a yearly basis was not great as compared to those done in clinics outside the community, but the number of requests was unquestionably large. During one year, for example, the local newspaper reported that approximately 1,100 local women had had abortions somewhere in the state; 57 percent, or 641, had been performed in Daleton hospitals. (The number of in-office abortions was not reported.) Abortion clinics assumed a major role because in principle they were known for not refusing requests. Although cost may be cited as a crucial factor in many women's decisions about where they go for abortions, no Daleton physician reduced the fee for this service in order to compete with the clinics. Certainly an opportunity to make money existed. And in that sense, the unwillingness to reduce fees may have followed from the expectation that demand would be great.

In the specialized clinic setting, the physician did not acquire the reputation of performing abortions; the *clinic* did. When referrals for abortion were made outside the community, they were made to clinics, not to specific physicians. The institution of private practice appeared less conducive to the provision of abortion services, perhaps because of the association of the particular physician with the services offered. No physician in Daleton listed abortion as a specialty in the yellow pages of the telephone book.[11] This further suggested how doctors avoided being associated with some of the services they provided. In the same telephone book, the three listings for birth control services outside the community contained no physicians' names but did describe specific services provided (for example, abortion).

If complaints were made about the assembly-line character of abortion clinic services, they stemmed, in part, from the de-emphasis on *who* gave the service. This impersonality produced its own form of discreetness for both physicians and patients. At the same time, the higher prices charged in the private practice setting served the interests of patients who preferred a private doctor to a public clinic and of doctors who preferred to be known publicly as obstetrician/gynecologists rather than abortionists. Even the most liberal physicians were sensitive to the importance of their reputations. The successful practice of medicine in a community required recognition and approval from patients and colleagues. If there was a public preference for discreet abortion services, it was served equally well by physicians who performed them but managed not to be known for performing them and by clinics outside the community.

The Younger Practitioners and the Conflict of Convictions

Physicians between thirty and forty years old had completed residency during the time when liberalization of abortion laws occurred. For a number of years after 1973, residents at Daleton Hospital were expected to learn how to perform abortions. One year, however, several of them complained to attendings about this policy. The attendings, all of whom were obstetrician/gynecologists in private practice, agreed to perform them if the residents objected.

In the larger community of Daleton, at approximately the same time that residents asked to be excused from performing abortions, disputes began between Planned Parenthood and United Way over funding for abortions through the local clinic. As mentioned in the last chapter, the United Way's decision to suspend funding to Planned Parenthood if it continued to offer abortion services appeared to force a change of policy at Daleton Hospital, where these services were always given. Physicians at the hospital indicated that the controversy depicted in the newspaper was incidental to the fact that, as attendings, they had agreed earlier not to "expect" residents to perform abortions. With the loss of funds from Planned Parenthood to subsidize the costs of the procedure, referrals to the clinics became more common.

Younger doctors in private practice in Daleton offered the most personal accounts about their changing attitudes toward abortion. Their wives figured prominently in their reasons for avoiding the procedure as much as possible. One doctor who had trained at Daleton during this time explained that he had been "involved in pregnancy terminations as a young resident" but that he and his wife, after talking it over, had decided that it was now against their "moral and religious feelings" for him to continue to do so. Another doctor who had regularly performed abortions during residency and for a while in private practice was now referring patients to the clinics. He admitted that he and his wife, who was Catholic, had avoided the subject: "It was never a big topic in the house and she is happy that I don't do them any more. In our own marriage we have had infertility problems and my wife could never see me doing abortions with our own problems being the way they were."

The changed context of medical practice for younger physicians can be seen another way in a cross-tabulation of their willingness to perform elective abortions with the degree of religiosity (as measured by church attendance) they professed. Table 4.1 shows that a high degree of religiosity correlated significantly with a physician's unwillingness to perform elective abortions. For six others who refused to do the procedure, religiosity did not appear to be a principal factor in their decision. Two of these were Protestants in a group that had decided collectively to refuse such requests. One was Jewish, an older solo practitioner. The remaining three who refused, two Protestants and one Jew, had come from residency programs in major urban settings, where there was a great demand for abortions. One of these

Table 4.1 | Cross-Tabulation of Church Attendance and Willingness to Perform Elective Abortions

	Regularly	Infrequently	Never
Yes	0% (0)	60% (3) P(2) + J(1)	70% (7) P(5) + J(1) + C(1)
Performs electives			
No	100% (9) C(5) + P(3) + J(1)	40% (3) P(2) + J(1)	30% (3) P(2) + J(1)

Note: The one Catholic physician not interviewed is not included in this table. J = Jewish, P = Protestant, C = Catholic.

three, Dr. Douglas, had actively participated as a resident in numerous outpatient abortions. He remarked that throughout training his wife had been upset about his performing them: "My wife is very strict anti-abortion. She believes the fetus has a personal right to exist. She's been a lot happier since we moved here." His wife was pleased, he said, because he had joined a group that referred all elective requests for abortion elsewhere. He was no longer bound by the expectations of attendings and thus was able to reconcile his wife's beliefs with his medical practice. He did not rule out the possibility of some day performing an abortion for a patient. But by developing a busy obstetrical practice, he knew that the probability of being asked to perform one would be reduced significantly.

A second physician, Dr. Pearlman, had done his residency at a large urban teaching hospital in the Northeast. His arrival in Daleton marked a dramatic change in the kinds of work he did in obstetrics and gynecology:

> I did many many abortions as a resident, first and second trimesters. But I find abortions disconcerting. At [the hospital where he did his residency] we used to get women coming in, one said to me, and this finished it for me, she said, "Hey, boy, wait on me, I don't want to be pregnant." . . . I don't engage in abortions here. I don't enjoy doing them. It is legalized murder, which has a place in society, but Ob/Gyn is antithetical to committing murder. There are rare mitigating circumstances, such as rape or incest, or a patient I have known. I don't know when life *is*, but quite frankly, hands and arms [of a fetus] are just that. I'm a right-to-lifer who believes in abortion.

Learning to perform abortions had been considered a legitimate and important part of becoming an obstetrician/gynecologist. Dr. Pearlman remarked that "if you were not Catholic, you were given little choice but to learn these techniques" because of the tremendous demand for this service in urban areas.

If such pressures to perform abortions did exist in some residency programs, the move into private practice permitted a much broader discretion about what to do. Dr. Pearlman now referred all requests for abortions to other members of his group. His reasoning about when the procedure was indicated was determined less by his training than by the fact that he was in private practice. He could now freely interpret his responsibilities and could define the "medical" needs of a patient requesting an abortion in any way he chose. From his new perspective, the "rare mitigating circumstances" that would compel him to perform the procedure could range from rape or incest to a request from "a patient I have known."

As illogical as this reasoning appeared, it was sociologically consistent with Dr. Pearlman's move away from the culture of clinics (including his and other residency programs) and into private practice. Outside the culture of clinics, he reinvented criteria that justified the distinction between an elective and a therapeutic abortion. His rationale for performing the procedure did not focus on its technical safety, as was more the case for Dr. Simpson, but on whether there were justifications for it in his mind. And as was typical for many doctors in Daleton, the request for an abortion seemed more legitimate coming from a patient who was known to him than from one who was not.

Like Dr. Douglas and Dr. Pearlman, Dr. Vincent of group three had acquired considerable skill in a variety of abortion techniques before coming to Daleton. After completing his residency, he had taught for several years at a major urban hospital located in a ghetto area of a large city in the Northeast. Before taking up his practice in Daleton, he informed the other members of his group that he would no longer perform abortions: "I came to my residency [in 1969] very pro-abortion. I still am in a way, except that I prefer not doing them any more. I remember the trouble my mother had getting a sterilization. They continually refused to give it to her. So I understand the problems of those in the lower socio-economic groups." Dr. Vincent's father, a plumber, and his mother, a waitress, had not finished high school. Although he was no longer formally religious, he had been active in the Methodist Church while growing up and had considered going into the ministry as a teenager. This early calling was perhaps reflected in his willingness to ponder and discuss his changing commitment to abortion and the practice of medicine.[12]

Before coming to Daleton, Dr. Vincent regularly performed abortions past the first trimester:

> Most of the abortions we did involved patients who did not use contraception. We were doing a lot of second-trimester abortions, and I thought I was doing a service. But not knowing the patients and not seeing them in any follow-up made me feel badly about doing them. We used a suction machine for the second-trimester abortion [a procedure known as a D & E, dilation and evacuation [13]]. What we did involved going in, crushing the skull, and pulling out pieces. I came to the conclusion I was killing babies. I feel it's a dilemma, it's emotionally distasteful. If I have any relationship with the patient, I will not say no, but I do feel a little less than honorable about doing them. It's disgusting pulling out arms and legs. It was a traumatic experience being involved in them. I have only done two in the past year and a half, and I hope not to be involved at all in this practice.

As is described in more detail in the next chapter, methods for second-trimester abortion evoked strong expressions of uncertainty among many physicians who otherwise accepted the procedure in the first trimester.

Dr. Vincent further remarked: "If my wife and I had an unwanted pregnancy, we would never have an abortion." But his wife's beliefs about the right to abortion were very strong, and for a time she was disappointed by his unwillingness to practice what he (or she) preached:

> She didn't understand my original difficulties. When I would come home and say, "Geez, I'm not comfortable doing this"—she didn't understand that, because again, politically she would say, "How can you believe this politically and then say you don't feel that you can do this?" She didn't understand that. She wasn't doing them and she didn't understand what that feeling was.

Whether or not their wives approved of their performing abortions, Daleton's younger physicians often spoke of the important role their spouses played in their decisions about how to practice medicine. Some wives were happy that their husbands had found a community and a medical practice in which the demand for abortion could be met by someone else. Those who more actively supported family planning were less satisfied with their husbands' decisions to avoid work in abortion. Caught between the pressures of home and community as well as between conviction and practice, these physicians, such as Dr. Vincent and Dr. Ingram, took refuge in their private practices. They were also among the most articulate about the impact of family, colleagues, patients, and community on the practice of medicine.

Because Dr. Vincent was one of the last physicians interviewed, I told him that I had met two others (that is, Dr. Pearlman and Dr. Douglas) who had also been actively trained to perform abortions during residency and who looked upon Daleton (and the private-practice setting) as an escape from those earlier experiences. He proceeded to jot down the names of two colleagues at his former hospital who were now in private practice and who, like him, were no longer performing abortions as much as they had. He offered to have his former secretary send me their telephone numbers. In the same breath he insisted that he did not want to impose his personal feelings or experiences on others. Yet he wondered how this was possible to avoid "when telling a woman you do not perform abortions." He was relieved by the knowledge that he could refer such cases to his partners in group three.

In this chapter and in chapter 3, I attempt to depict some of the factors that influenced physicians' decisions to agree or refuse to perform abortions. Certain ascribed features, such as age and religion, were significant for how they defined their responsibilities toward family planning. When and where they received their medical training had consequences for how they chose to practice obstetrics and gynecology once in private practice. The structure of private practice itself afforded innumerable strategies to reconcile personal beliefs with medical responsibilities. Finally, between family and home on the one side and profession and community on the other, physicians in private practice were able to respond to requests for abortion as they saw fit.

In preferring not to be known as local abortionists, several physicians acknowledged the constraints of practicing medicine in a community. Family planning advocates blamed Daleton's "conservative climate" for physicians' reluctance to open a specialized clinic for abortion. In sociological terms, this reluctance was institutionally supported by the structure of private practice and professionally reinforced by the special demands placed on the practitioner to establish a competence that was specialized, but not narrow.

The types of clinical work physicians chose to do in Daleton did not always depend on their experiences in that community. The youngest and most skilled technicians of abortion, trained outside Daleton, had purposely chosen to discontinue their clinical work with it. As the newest members of the community, they knew least about Daleton's family planning politics. In their previous clinical community—that is, in residency—they were expected to conform to what Charles Bosk has described as the norms and "quasi-norms" of their superordinates (1979:51–67). Training conformity was superseded by the various constraints of practicing in a community.[14] The opinions of the physicians' wives in some cases influenced their approaches to abortion. In place of the normative constraints of medical training, the decision to perform an abortion in private practice was discussed not only with the patient or with colleagues but also in the context of a marriage. Perhaps no clearer evidence existed that abortion touched upon the professional *and* personal lives of many of the physicians in this community. As routine and safe as it had become, it symbolized the dilemma about the physician's medical responsibility to all who requested his expertise or who sought to influence it.

The inconsistencies in physicians' rationales for agreeing or refusing to perform abortions underscored the unusual nature of this medical responsibility. Avoidance of abortion, particularly by those best trained to perform it, appeared to violate professional standards which demanded that the best possible care be given, but it affirmed an even deeper expectation about the privileges afforded physicians in private practice. Of course, the physician's privilege not to perform an abortion placed a constraint on the right of a woman to have one performed. In the minds of many doctors, the abortion clinic had become the logical response to this constraint. It represented the institutionalization of abortion that the private practice of medicine, however unintentionally, resisted. The organization of resistance to abortion had other features, not least of which was the physician's acknowledgment of what was aborted.

5
The Second-Trimester Abortion: Limited Procedures

The limit is still twenty weeks, because you're still getting the twenty-two-weekers at twenty weeks. All you have to do is go a little bit further and you're talking about viability, as they have survivors at twenty-four weeks. So you up your limit to say twenty-two weeks, then you're going to have the occasional twenty-four-weeker. Kind of the standard of the community as far as defining life is when a fetus can live. I will not violate the standards of the community.

Dr. Hill

Termination of pregnancy beyond the twelfth week has been less easily routinized than termination during the first trimester, in part because different technical approaches are required. Until the demand for this procedure increased following the legalization of abortion in 1973, one frequently used method called for injection of hypertonic saline solution directly into the amniotic sac. After many hours, the action of the salt solution causes expulsion of the fetus. This method is particularly hazardous between the thirteenth and fifteenth weeks (Bolognese and Corson, 1975:126). At that stage of fetal development, the fetus and the amniotic sac are not easily separated and removed. Physicians who used saline waited until after the sixteenth week to proceed.

During the past ten years, extensive work has been done with prostaglandins, several of which have been clinically demonstrated to cause abortion "by inducing uterine activity physiologically similar to that of normal labor" (ibid.,

77

p. 110). One form of prostaglandin "appears to exert a definite re-laxing effect on the cervix," thereby making delivery of the uterine contents easier to accomplish (p. 125). Prostaglandins can be administered in at least three ways: by intravenous infusion, by direct injection into the uterus between the fetal membrane and the uterine wall (known as extraovular drug administration), and by vaginal suppositories. They have been shown to work in first- and second-trimester abortions; one advantage they have over the saline method, especially during the thirteenth to fifteenth weeks, is that they need not be injected directly into the amniotic sac.

With all the methods utilizing saline or prostaglandins, the time from the administration of the treatment to the induction of labor and finally to the expulsion of the uterine contents can range from several hours to several days, depending on the particular method, the length of gestation, the drug dosage, and other factors. On average, the entire process takes between twelve and twenty-four hours. The routinization of any medical service includes the actual time required to give it as well as its cost. With prostaglandins, the time factor has contributed to a decline in its acceptance as the preferred method, and the requirement of hospitalization raises its cost considerably. Side effects associated with saline and prostaglandin techniques have also been cited as a discouragement to their wide use. "Vomiting and/or diarrhea is the most common side effect occurring in 55% to 85% of patients" receiving prostaglandins (Bolognese and Corson, 1975:143; see also Corson et al., 1973, and Zatuchni et al., 1979).[1] The least preferred method of termination beyond the first trimester is hysterotomy, or what is sometimes called a mini-Cae-sarean section. As it is the most invasive surgery, it carries the highest risks of morbidity and mortality.

In recent years, a combination technique (D & E, or dilation and evacuation) using conventional curettage and vacuum aspiration has been employed as an effective method. Although medical complications are likely to increase with any method used in the second trimester, one advantage of D & E is that termination is completed as soon as the operation is performed. Saline- and prostaglandin-induced abortions require more time, and studies report that they cause greater discomfort and stress to the patient (Berger et al., 1981). The growing acceptance of D & E over the other methods signals its routinization; it takes less time, it is less expensive, and side effects are not as uncertain as with prostaglandins. Dilation and evacuation rarely requires extended hospitalization, and it is now increasingly performed in abortion facilities across the United States on an out-patient basis.

Despite this progress, abortions after the first trimester have retained an experimental character that has made them medically interesting for some physicians but medically problematic for others. Techniques for second-trimester abortions were standardized first in places where they were most often requested and performed. The diffusion of what is considered standard in the case of this procedure has largely depended on the results of epidemiological studies that have shown the superior effectiveness and safety of D & E over all other methods.[2]

Without the sustained scrutiny of such government agencies as the Abortion Surveillance Division of the Federal Centers for Disease Control, medical consensus about second-trimester abortion techniques would not have formed so rapidly. Routinization was thus accelerated by systematic reporting from major providers of the service. Statistical studies demonstrated the effectiveness and safety of D & E, but researchers also noted that the method was less time-consuming for patients and staff.

The reduction of time was not the only factor contributing to the improved service to patients. With saline and prostaglandins, patients were also subjected to the experience of labor, and nurses were often expected (in lieu of a physician) to preside over the "delivery." In reporting on a symposium sponsored in 1981 under the auspices of the National Abortion Federation, Sarah Lewit of the Population Council concluded:

> The symposium left no doubt that with D & E procedures, the psychological burden was lifted from the patients and the nurses with whom it had been left under the instillation regimen and shifted to the physicians, who henceforth must rely ". . . on a strong sense of social conscience which focused on the health and desires of the women." (1982:54)[3]

The appeal to a "strong sense of social conscience" among doctors was reminiscent of the call to "serve the new society in which we live" made by one hundred professors of obstetrics in a manifesto to the profession in 1972 ("A Statement on Abortion by One Hundred Professors of Obstetrics," 1972:992). The shift in responsibility, which imposed new expectations upon doctors once abortion was legalized, was repeated in the extramedical justifications given to support innovations in abortion techniques.

The statistically "safer" technology did not eliminate the "psychological burden" associated with second-trimester abortion but only shifted it. Epidemiological surveillance was useful for clarifying what medical complications occurred. If the complications associated with prostaglandins, for instance, could have been further reduced by instituting appropriate monitoring and treatments, more than a residue of the psychological burden of having to deliver the fetus would have remained. Shifting the psychological burden to the physician could not be justified on scientific, much less medical, grounds alone. It is clear that those advocating D & E were also appealing to the sensibilities of physicians who presumably could be persuaded to take on more of the responsibility for removing the fetus. In the context of private practice, physician judgment about how to proceed was paramount. In Daleton, physicians avoided professing their social consciences or facing psychological burdens. Instead, they referred abortion requests beyond the first trimester to Dr. Hill.

I first met with Dr. Hill on the fifth floor of Daleton Hospital, where the maternity ward is located. He asked me to wait in the "fathers' waiting room." When he arrived, he was in surgical dress, a green face mask still draped around his neck. His responses to our first interview were straightforward, brief, and occasionally sarcastic. Although his opinion of the American Medical Association was shared by many other physicians in the community, his feelings were more strongly stated: "I do not have many positive reasons for being a member. They continue to condone incompetence in physicians. They do not support strong educational requirements in medical schools, and they are definitely unable to fight off the government. They are really just a political organization." Dr. Hill had no contact with Planned Parenthood; he explained that at Daleton Hospital only residents did and that he had not done his residency there. He claimed to have been the first resident at his residency hospital to perform a first-trimester abortion, for the "niece of the head of my department, who was in a family way." A therapeutic abortion committee in that hospital in 1967 approved the abortion for "social reasons."

Although he never refused to perform an abortion for a woman requesting one, "I make people go home and think it over." In his private practice, he attributed 30 percent of the abortions he performed to contraceptive failure and 70 percent to a lack of sex education; the latter he thought was "really gross." He believed that "proper sex education would take care of it." Contraceptive failure represented a technical problem that called for innovations in technique. He hoped that technical imperfections would some day be eliminated, and he argued that sex education was a problem well beyond the specific medical duties of the physician.

Dr. Hill performed between 30 and 50 abortions a year in the second trimester. His willingness to perform them was best explained by the way he perceived the role of the physician in the public controversy over abortion: "To prohibit abortions would lead again to kitchen-table abortions and ladies dying. I don't think the physician needs to be any part of the controversy. The physician is just a technician." He did not distinguish between elective and therapeutic abortion when deciding whether to perform the procedure. However, a story he told showed that he was willing to accommodate a patient who preferred one abortion technique over another:

> I had a Catholic woman who was guilty as hell about having an abortion and who knew something about [abortion] techniques. She wanted me to perform a D & C [for an early second-trimester abortion, between twelve and thirteen weeks] rather than use a prostaglandin because for her the D & C only removed some tissue, while the prostaglandin delivered a whole fetus. So I did the D & C which at the time was definitely more difficult and less safe for me to do, because for her it entailed only the removing of tissue, not a fetus. I think it is illogical, but then, who am I to judge? Her relief will far outweigh the guilt.

For several years, he worked extensively with prostaglandins. His willingness to accommodate this patient's request was based on the belief that he could perform either technique safely enough, though he admitted that in his medical judgment prostaglandins were safer and more effective. But the margin of safety between the two was not large enough to outweigh his patient's moral reservations. The only moral issue in his opinion was the relative danger of abortion under legal and illegal circumstances. His choice of method in this case did not depend upon the status of the fetus. He would take the matter of viability more seriously in the case of late second-trimester abortions (for example, around 20 weeks).

If he had any reservations about performing abortions, Dr. Hill expressed them more in terms of medical probabilities than in a concern for the fetus:

> I don't think that the attitudes of a woman can be understood by men. They have a logic which is impossible to fathom sometimes. I had a lady who wanted an abortion because she was soon going to be in a horse show and couldn't fit into her riding outfit. She got pregnant again four months later, but I though the whole thing was stupid since any pregnancy has its danger, and why risk it a second time if you don't have to? But who am I to judge?

At the conclusion of our first meeting, we shook hands, and he said:

> What you really ought to be studying are the attitudes of women who have their own minds about these things which men could never hope to understand.

As the technician par excellence of abortion, Dr. Hill saw his approach to the procedure as entirely rational. He attributed all irrationality in the resort to abortion to women patients, who exhibited "a logic which is impossible to fathom sometimes." By responding twice, "Who am I to judge?" he expressed no personal reservations about performing the procedure for any reason. This does not mean that he found all reasons understandable, especially from a medical point of view.

Dr. Hill's remarks about patients were at the same time condescending and respectful; he noticed but disregarded their motives and responded technically as well as he could to their requests for services. Conceding that he did not believe abortion was the best way to control birth, he nevertheless considered each patient's request in practical rather than abstract terms. He said that he often asked patients to "think it over," and to this extent he was more honest with them about *his* motives than were many of his colleagues who used referrals as a way of meeting their professional duties while avoiding direct involvement.

A Catholic member of Dr. Hill's group remarked that he had more than once tried to dissuade his colleague from performing second-trimester abortions. He knew about Dr. Bernard Nathanson, the

New York physician who had resigned as head of an abortion clinic and had publicly stated his misgivings in the *New England Journal of Medicine:* "I hoped for my partner after I read about him [Nathanson]. It shows a guy has guts enough to swing 180 degrees around the other way." Dr. Hill was aware of his partner's concerns. He pointed out that they got along well because they had agreed "to practice medicine and not politics" in their group.

The perception of Dr. Hill among his colleagues and in the larger community confirmed that he was both highly respected and controversial. His surgical abilities were praised by physicians on staff at Daleton Hospital, and he was known to accept difficult cases, such as second-trimester abortions. Attempts had been made to "discredit" him early in his practice (in the early 1970s). One of his colleagues in another group remarked that Dr. Hill was "known to have a sign hanging in his office which reads 'You Fuck 'Em, We Suck 'Em.' " In a follow-up interview with Dr. Hill (after he had read portions of my manuscript describing his colleagues' opinions), he responded sardonically to the allegation:

> The physician that told you about the sign hanging in my office—I didn't think [he mentioned the physician's first name] was one of my discreditors. He's just a character like I am. I would never place him on a list of somebody trying to discredit me. Discredit came from other quarters. We had to send a letter to a Catholic priest a few years ago. He used my name from the pulpit. Threatened to sue. That stopped that.

Dr. Hill reaffirmed a stereotypical view about the fraternity of doctors. Discredit came from outside the profession, not from within.

Over the five years that I spent broadly monitoring Daleton doctors, only one incident occurred in which a physician, an oncologist on staff at St. Timothy, was censured by the local medical society. He was accused of having made false claims about the outcomes of reconstructive breast surgery following mastectomy. By granting an interview to a local reporter, he caused a small panic among women patients of other physicians in the community who had not performed the same kind of procedure. An editorial in the journal of the local medical society severely criticized him for raising false hopes about surgery for carcinoma of the breast. Already on the periphery of the professional community of physicians (for example, he was not a member of the medical society and was on staff at the least prestigious hospital in Daleton), he was easily discredited for his claims about scientifically unconfirmed results. Dr. Hill, on staff at the most prestigious hospital and respected for his medical work by his colleagues, was less susceptible to being professionally maligned. Innuendo about the abortions he performed was the only discredit he suffered.

Dr. Hill regularly performed first- and second-trimester abortions at Daleton Hospital. Unlike several of his colleagues, he did not express concern about his reputation in the larger community. His sense of reputation did not depend on what he was known to do but on whether he was known to do it well. To him the charge of "abortionist" implied professional incompetence. He saw no relationship between public attacks on his abortion practices and loss of status in the professional community. A prestigious hospital setting combined with a highly respected group practice diminished the stigma of abortionist. Yet these social sources of reputation were strengthened by his personal resolve to respond publicly (for example, by hiring a lawyer) to charges made against him. Other physicians had achieved prominent reputations in the larger community by effectively concealing their abortion practices from everyone but their closest patients. Private practice mediated between two sources of reputation: one's colleagues and the larger community. Dr. Hill earned the respect of colleagues despite his abortion practices, while other doctors achieved standing in the larger community by being known for other services.

Besides Dr. Hill, only Dr. Roth, on staff at St. Timothy, was known to perform abortions beyond the first trimester. Dr. Roth was unwilling to talk at length about his abortion practices, but Dr. Hill suggested several reasons why this solo practitioner preferred to maintain a low profile in the community. In the first place, Dr. Roth's primary affiliation was with a Catholic hospital. He performed abortions during the afternoons at Central. Dr. Hill revealed that Dr. Roth had also been allowed to perform second-trimester abortions at Daleton Hospital. When I remarked that Dr. Roth would not talk with me about abortion, Dr. Hill replied:

Well, he doesn't talk to anybody. But he brought a patient over [to Daleton Hospital] who was twenty-four weeks. That kind of upset the girls in the delivery room up to the point where I had to write him a letter and present the standards of the community to him, and asked that he kindly not do that again. Because as I understand it, he did a few at Central, and they asked him not to do them down there again for the same reason. And I'm not saying he can't do them here, but he has got to take into consideration the sensibilities of the people around him.

While performing late second-trimester abortions with prostaglandins at Central Hospital, Dr. Roth had encountered similar difficulties with the supporting staff. When I asked Dr. Hill whether Dr. Roth regularly performed second-trimester abortions, he responded:

> No. He just does an occasional one. I didn't even know he did them until that patient came up. Of course, bad word kind of travels fast. The girls in the delivery room found out that he wasn't allowed to do them at Central any more. I really don't go noseying around. I have enough work to do just to work. The only reason I found out about this was because the chief of OB asked me to please write him [Dr. Roth] a letter, because I did all these [second-trimester abortions] over here. So I did. It was signed by the director of the Department of OB and myself.

Dr. Roth conducted his medical practice in a manner that drew little attention to himself, except for "the girls in the delivery room." It was the offense to the "sensibilities of the people around him" in the operating room, not his colleagues, that called the "standards of the community" to the attention of other physicians.

The formal letter sent by the physicians to Dr. Roth did not prohibit him from performing abortions at Daleton Hospital, but the strong disapproval of supporting staff in effect deterred him from performing late second-trimester ones there. Dr. Roth's use of prostaglandins upset the supporting staff for two reasons, according to Dr. Hill. First, Dr. Roth had expected the staff to cope with the delivery, and second, by performing the abortions so late, he had offended the sensibilities of those who worked with him and who knew that the prospects of delivering viable infants increased significantly after twenty-four weeks.

The formal censure of Dr. Roth was the outcome of interactions he had with the supporting staff. In this regard, Dr. Hill had a distinct advantage over his colleague in that he was a staff member of the hospital. Just as physicians were more likely to accept requests for first-trimester abortions from patients whom they knew, so the supporting staff at Daleton Hospital was more willing to participate in second-trimester abortions when performed by a physician whom they knew. Dr. Hill had earned their confidence; Dr. Roth threatened that confidence by expecting them to participate in ways that Dr. Hill had sought to avoid.

Dr. Hill remarked that when he first began using prostaglandins for pregnancy termination, during his residency, he occasionally saw "live births." He referred to live birth as a possible "side effect of prostaglandins." He had witnessed deliveries of fetuses that had "detectable heartbeats and had tried to gasp." These "side effects" initially discouraged him about the effectiveness of this new method. For a time he used combinations of hypertonic glucose and hypertonic saline solutions. One technical advantage of this method was that the saline solution acted as a caustic agent, destroying the fetus in utero.

By the mid-1970s, Dr. Hill was working exclusively with prostaglandins, and he had developed ways to avoid the delivery of fetuses that exhibited any signs of life. He instructed his nurses to tell the patient not to push after the injection of the prostaglandin, thus keeping the fetus in utero long enough to be aborted without any signs of life. By doing this, he explained, "I don't have these [that is, live birth] problems." By the early 1980s, after many years of experimenting with prostaglandins, he had settled on using D & E up to seventeen weeks of gestation:

> The patients prefer it that way. The only problem is a personnel problem. It's an unattractive method because you have to morselate [that is, cut into small pieces] the fetus, and then remove it with forceps rather than a nice little suction catheter. The girls in the operating room don't exactly draw straws to go in with you. But that's a minor problem. The way people usually do the prostaglandins is not the way I usually did them. So I don't think my morbidity is going to change much [with D & E]. But when they demonstrated that it was at least as safe, if not safer, than [prostaglandins], the differences in cost to the patient and to the insurance company makes it a matter of selecting the cost-effective way, and that's D & E. It's just an ambulatory surgical procedure versus a two- or three-day hospitalization.

Second-trimester abortions presented Dr. Hill and Dr. Roth with technical difficulties and appeared to cause some discontent among supporting staff regardless of the procedure used.

One physician who had worked with second-trimester methods

in a residency outside Daleton remarked that he had a responsibility to his colleagues as well as to his supporting staff: "In a group practice, I couldn't subject my colleagues to taking care of something I had started [for example, injection of prostaglandins], if for some reason I couldn't be there. Of course there would be no problem with normal deliveries, but other physicians in a group practice might not want to be involved in any part of a second-trimester abortion."

Dr. Vincent, one of Dr. Hill's partners, had also performed second-trimester abortions outside Daleton. His descriptions of that work (chap. 4) were among the most vivid expressed by any physician I interviewed. He strongly defended Dr. Hill's right to perform second-trimester abortions and said he would not object to supervising a prostaglandin-induced delivery if his partner were unavailable. But he could no longer imagine doing such an injection himself. His rationale, it should be noted, was based on a sense of professional responsibility. He could not perform the injection, but he held himself medically responsible for the patient's health regardless of the circumstances.

The two criteria for determining the best method for second-trimester abortions were the relative safety of the procedure (as shown by epidemiological studies) and its cost-effectiveness. Regardless of the method used, however, the achievement of maximum safety and cost-effectiveness could not conceal the doctor's recognition of what was aborted. The avoidance of second-trimester abortions by the majority of physicians in Daleton was partly the result of uncertainty about whether one was aborting or delivering a potentially viable fetus.

The determination of viability was once a matter for obstetric jurisprudence and forensic medicine.[4] The word *viability* is mentioned in the 1940 edition of Bland and Montgomery's *Practical Obstetrics,* but the notion is more clearly addressed in their attempt to define under what circumstances the destruction of a fetus/infant could be medically and legally termed infanticide:

A live birth is usually predicated on the evidence of the occurrence of respiration, though it must be recalled that children may for some time after birth show no signs of breathing at all. In some children respiration may be brought about by artificial means and they may survive.(1940:814)

In cases of suspected infanticide, the pathologist was called in to establish whether the child had breathed. In 1975, Dr. Richard E. Behrman and Dr. Tove S. Rosen offered the following definition of *viability*, which exhibited important differences when compared to the 1940 definition of *live birth:*

> A fetus or prematurely delivered infant is biologically viable when a minimal number of independently sustained, basic, integrative physiological functions are present. In order for the fetus or infant to be viable the sum of these functions, considered together, must support the inference that the fetus or premature infant is able to increase in tissue mass (growth) and increase the number, complexity, and coordination of basic physiologic functions (development) as a self-sustaining whole organism. This must be independent of any connection with the mother and when receiving only generally accepted medical treatments. If, in sum, these coordinated functions are not present, the fetus or prematurely born infant is biologically nonviable since it is incapable of being made able to exist as a self-sustaining whole organism independently of any connection with the mother. This may be the case even though some signs of life are apparent. (1975:12–25)

The 1940 definition stressed that respiration "may be brought about by artificial means," even when signs of respiratory function are not present. On the other hand, the 1975 definition concluded that viability may not be present "even though some signs of life are apparent." The difference between the two definitions reflected progress in diagnostic and technological medicine; by 1975, signs of life not previously apparent could be detected.

After the legalization of abortion, viability marked the point at which a physician was expected to act on behalf of a fetus. The use of fetuses for experimental purposes also called for a working rather than theoretical definition of when the preservation of life was to take precedence over scientific research. The criteria for viability in 1975 were stated in probabilities and were intended to guide scientific understanding of when a fetus became a biologically independent being. In 1940, the evidence sought was of a unique, particularistic, and retrospective sort: Was respiration evident, and if not, could it have been brought about by artificial means?

The increased availability and use of artificial means of life support complicated the problem of reconciling theoretical definitions of viability with practical recommendations about how to proceed medically. The probability of viability had been increased by medical technology in many cases of premature delivery. In place of the courts, the physician was left to determine the probability of viability, depending on the abortion technique used and the medical resources (for example, artificial means of life support) available. The preference for use of D & E in second-trimester abortions, especially over prostaglandins, reflected the aim of destroying the fetus and thereby avoiding what might otherwise be taken for a premature delivery. From this perspective, in the case of a late second-trimester abortion, the use of prostaglandins was the least desirable method.

The conflict between theory and practice was epitomized in physicians' responses to the definition of viability. The Supreme Court in its 1973 rulings had followed conventional medical wisdom by repeating that viability occurred during the third trimester. Most physicians in Daleton, for example, defined viability in terms of fetal weight (roughly 500 grams) and length of gestation (twenty-eight weeks). To the extent that it was supposed to mark the time limit for an elective abortion, viability had become an equivocal concept in the law. With different abortion techniques available and with different opinions about when artificial life supports should be applied, viability was determined more by the actions of physicians in the contexts of their medical practices than by probabilistic estimates of physiological growth.[5]

One physician who put viability at twenty-eight weeks was reluctant to speculate on what would happen if technologies that could artificially sustain fetal life during the second trimester were to become widely available. He concluded, "I prefer to deal with what is, not with what can be." His unwillingness to perform second-trimester abortions, though he was not opposed to them, was due to the "trickiness of the procedures involved." Because of these technical difficulties, he believed that such abortions should be performed regularly by those who were experienced in doing them. In the face of recognizable complications of a medical, legal, and moral kind, he invoked his privilege to practice as he saw fit: "I have morally no feelings about it one way or the other. It is the kind of thing I suppose which is generally repugnant, but I don't have to make the moral decision."

Dr. Simpson of group one, who regularly performed elective first-trimester abortions, candidly admitted why he did not as a rule perform them in the second trimester:

> Look, Jonathan, I have one hell of a big practice. I need no glory. Of course anywhere between twelve and twenty-four weeks, if it is truly indicated, that is if there are sound logical, medical reasons for me to do it, say, genetic reasons, well then, yes, I'll do it. But just because she came in here eighteen weeks pregnant, I don't need her. . . . I've never had a medical-legal problem. Some young guy who needs the money, he can take the risk. Second-trimester terminations are bad from the medical-legal point of view.

One of Dr. Simpson's older partners referred to second-trimester abortions as "salting-outs," the colloquial medical expression for hypertonic saline-induced abortions. His definition of viability revealed his own taxonomic uncertainties: "I'm not sure I can answer that for myself: A child, er, a fetus which—notice I said which—is capable of living without the uterine environment. If I say who, I automatically assume it's a person. By implication, I would call it a person."

Another doctor who at one time had regularly performed elective abortions put viability at twenty-eight weeks but reported that he had delivered several infants at less than twenty-six weeks who had survived. An elective request for an abortion had temporal limits in his view: "The information I've seen indicates that they wish to have the pregnancy continue if they let it go that long. By that point they realize they are pregnant. Maybe I feel they should feel this way. In any case I have to pick a point at which I would be uncomfortable performing an abortion." This response captured the prevailing ethos among Daleton physicians (other than Dr. Hill and Dr. Roth) about second-trimester abortions. A standard procedure became a limited one somewhere after the first trimester and before birth. In this temporal scheme, viability served as an outer limit. Yet, in practical terms, both the acknowledgment of fetal life and the need to use technically more complicated methods remained compelling factors that discouraged most physicians from performing abortions after the first trimester.

In the past ten years most states have promulgated regulations concerning the reporting of induced terminations of pregnancy.[6] At an earlier time, before the legalization and routinization of abortion, laws were passed that defined *live birth* and *fetal death*. Some states called for the issuance of birth and death certificates, depending on the gestational age and weight of the fetus. In the majority of states, the reporting of a "fetal death" was required if the fetus was more than twenty weeks or weighed more than 350 grams. A number of states also required a burial or removal permit for such fetuses. These requirements caused difficulties for physicians performing abortions in the second trimester. The bureaucratic requirements of birth and death certificates and of burial or licensed disposal discouraged Dr. Hill, for example, from performing abortions after twenty weeks.

The criteria of gestational age and weight were used interchangeably in some states, whereas other states required that only one or the other criterion had to be met for the issuance of birth and death certificates and burial. Daleton physicians were required to go by fetal age even though several of them insisted that it was sometimes difficult to determine exactly. One doctor, who responded in writing to my request for more information about these matters, described the consequences of his state's reporting requirements:

> I needn't tell you that this very archaic rule requiring birth and death certificates and burial for midtrimester pregnancies is a source of great concern, not only to the practitioner, but to the patient and her husband. The needless expense by the involvement of a mortician, which produces at least a $70.00 out-of-pocket expense for cremation, is burdensome to many couples; moreover, patients and husbands do not always seek this form of disposal, and with burial and a funeral service, the out-of-pocket expense is compounded many times, as you well know. The happy contrast of [a nearby state] quickly comes to mind. I refer many patients to [an out-of-state hospital] where, at 22, 23, or 24 weeks the clinical laboratory of the hospital is able to dispose of the pregnancy products, just as an amputated limb, or any other body tissue is disposed of in the laboratory incinerator.

Dr. Hill claimed that, as far as he knew, most other states did not require birth and death certificates for spontaneous or induced abortions of fetuses of less than 500 grams, or of less than twenty-four weeks' gestation. All his patients undergoing second-trimester abortions were asked to sign a form that gave the hospital the responsibility for disposing of the fetus. He made every effort to perform the abortions as early as possible, so that birth and death certificates and burial could be avoided. For very late second-trimester abortions, he too had decided to refer patients to another state, where these various bureaucratic difficulties did not exist.

A remarkable difference existed between the impact of state law on physicians' judgments about second-trimester abortions and that of the Supreme Court's 1973 rulings. The state and local rulings on the circumstances in which abortion could be made available were decidedly more conservative than the federal mandate. One physician quipped, "The Supreme Court doesn't know too much about biology." The Court permitted abortions "until viability," but not even Dr. Hill was willing to perform them past twenty weeks, and he preferred to do them before eighteen weeks. Medical consensus about abortions beyond the first trimester was shaped less by law than by developments in neonatal technology. After 1973, the new uncertainties created by these developments received public notice in several well-publicized cases in which physicians were prosecuted for performing second-trimester abortions on potentially viable fetuses.[7]

Dr. Robert E. Hall, who actively sought reform of state abortion laws prior to 1973, responded to the growing medical and public controversy about late-second-trimester abortions in a letter to the *New York Times* in February 1984:

> Advances in neonatology have intensified concern over fetuses' survival of abortion procedures, but they have not created the problem. It was always there.
>
> Prior to the Supreme Court's Roe v. Wade decision in 1973, an abortion was medically defined as the termination of a pregnancy before its 20th week, for even then there was known to be a small chance of fetal survival. In its otherwise laudable ruling, the Court erred in extending this deadline. Except in cases of known fetal deformity, the original, scientifically and morally defensible definition should be adhered to. The "advances in neonatology" argument may enable the Court to save face in rectifying its mistake. (1984:E18)[8]

The significance of Dr. Hall's letter was that it represented a return to medical standards that had been abandoned by the Court except in its mention of viability. Within the context of the politics of abortion, his assessment probably strengthened the position of the right-to-life movement. It was also a reminder that, beyond the politics of abortion, physician participation in abortion continued to be an important, if ignored, dimension in this larger political struggle, which appeared to offer no room for compromise. In reality, how physicians behaved with regard to abortion demonstrated the numerous compromises that were made every day in the practice of medicine, at least outside the culture of clinics.

In chapter 3, I have argued that physicians in private practice did not perform large numbers of abortions because of their low priority in terms of medical knowledge and operative technique. Board certification demanded more challenging approaches to treatment of disease and to surgical work. This conclusion would now appear to contradict the fact that most doctors were unwilling to perform second-trimester abortions precisely because of their technical challenge. But other medical and surgical challenges in obstetrics and gynecology were less controversial. In their efforts to avoid controversy, physicians in private practice scrutinized their relations with colleagues, patients, and the larger community. Their professional expectations about the value and efficacy of different forms of medical treatment were inseparable from those relations.

6
Innovation and the Refuge of Private Practice

The private practice of medicine allowed Daleton physicians to determine how they would handle requests for abortion. In this chapter, I move away from the specific issue of abortion in order to examine the nature of this practice in the lives of several of these doctors. By doing so, I intend to say more about the ways in which private practice served as the locus for innovation in their personal and professional commitments to patients. A physician's sense of vocation or calling to medicine created the grounds for innovation *within* private practice. On the other hand, the introduction of new medical treatments and technologies influenced how physicians assessed the risks and uncertainties of practicing medicine.

A physician's ability to control the process and outcome of medical work was shaped by the social nature of medical practice itself. Solo and group practices were formed for moral as well as economic reasons. The decision to join a group practice was often made initially as a matter of necessity, born of the expense of starting up a practice alone. Yet the decision to leave a group practice, whether to form another group practice or to practice alone, was sometimes the culmination of a doctor's long reflection about the aims of medical work. Physicians discussed the delivery of care in terms of their commitment to patients as well as in terms of their medical training and expertise. Their efforts to balance family life with medical practice, for example, showed that the commitment to that practice was more than a combination of skill and specialization; it also implicated many people around the doctor, including colleagues, family, and patients.

Innovation within Private Practice

A little more than three years after he joined group three, Dr. Vincent decided to move out on his own as a solo practitioner in obstetrics and gynecology. He had long considered the decision to move but actively pursued it following a number of disputes with his partners. Before coming to Daleton, he had been affiliated with a major urban teaching hospital where he had performed first- and second-trimester abortions. He announced to his partners in the Daleton group that he preferred not to perform abortions any more and would refer requests to them. About a year later another partner (who was not interviewed) was brought into the group.[1]

Dr. Vincent set up his new practice in offices previously occupied by another solo practitioner on staff at Daleton Hospital in a building owned by a group of dentists. When asked how his decision to move into solo practice came about, he first replied:

> I just decided I wanted to have my own practice and my absolute own patients. It's a big practice [that is, group three]. We did about 600 deliveries a year. And they were good people, good guys to work with. But I just felt that I wanted to call my own shots for me. And so I decided to do it. My partners think it's a mid-life crisis, but we're going to see. But that was the motivating factor.

Dr. Vincent's move from group to solo practice was counter to the national trend in the practice of obstetrics and gynecology. He was financially able to break away because he had many years of experience in both teaching and practicing.

In discussing the relative benefits of group and solo work, he noted the time that group practice had allowed him to spend with his family:

> My family and I spent a lot of time talking about it [that is, the move into solo practice], and just kind of felt that at this point in my life, it's what I needed to do for me. We've lived with me working on a regular on-call schedule every fourth night or so, and every fifth night up there [at the hospital], which has been very nice because I've had a lot of time

to be at home with my children and with my wife. That produces a very, very nice living situation as a physician. There's lots of free time, and I always had a day off a week.

But private time away from work was becoming less important now that his children were reaching their teenage years. He began to assess more carefully the quality of medical work and care in his group practice:

> I think that deep down inside my concept about medicine is that there is this agreement between you and the people you care for, that you'll be basically the person that doesn't end up in obstetrics with a big practice, six hundred people and five guys. You might only get to see people a couple of times. That's disappointing. It was neat to be involved in six hundred people's lives each year. That was exciting. But at times it was disappointing because there were people that I would have liked to be more involved with, but I just couldn't because of the way it works. So I wanted to try this to see how it is. And if it becomes too much, then I will probably take a partner or two, because I don't ever want to be in that big a group. I think that it loses some of the intimacy that women expect in a gynecologic practice.

Dr. Vincent had thought often about the benefits and drawbacks of a group's size. The "intimacy" he referred to was expressed in the sharing of knowledge and concern among his colleagues as much as between physician and patient.

He spoke of his experiences of doctoring in the form of anecdotes and reviewed incidents in his daily practice. He wanted to maintain good working relations with his partners, but his idea of good care also depended on his being informed about patients who were seen by other members of the group:

> What would happen sometimes would be you might see a patient—and you know with a busy practice maybe I'd see a hundred and fifteen people a week in three days, and I might be off that weekend—a patient that I had seen might have had some spotting or something, and it was conceivable that she could come in, be in early pregnancy, and either abort or have something else happen to her, have surgery, and leave. And I'd never know about it. I spent a lot of time talking with the guys about the need to share that information. Because you know that's not a question, amongst equals, of assuming that the care's not as good, but I have a bond to those people, too.

I can remember, not too long ago, with the youngest partner—the guy who had the smallest practice—that there was a patient who I had been following, who had some problems, and I had wanted to talk to her. She knew I'd be away on Sunday. I talked with her on Saturday. I wasn't on that weekend. I called her and she was doing okay. I came back on Monday and I called her to see how she was doing. She had come in Sunday morning and had miscarried and gone home. My partner never even told me, and he was working with me. That kind of thing disturbs me in the big group practice, because people then feel, and rightly so, that there is not a continuity.

Continuity was a moral as well as an organizational imperative. Dr. Vincent viewed its absence among his partners as the major structural flaw in the group, and he reported that he had talked with doctors in other groups who expressed similar reservations.

The benefits of group practice were intended for practitioner and patient alike. Dr. Vincent observed, "Groups exist so that the physicians can have free time, which is absolutely necessary in terms of being a human being." Group practice also provided for continuous coverage to patients, sometimes at the expense of communication among the partners. Dr. Vincent was troubled by this aspect of working in so large a group, even though he regarded his partners as "honorable, decent human beings." His complaint against the youngest partner might be construed as a conflict of personalities, or his partner's apparent indifference might be interpreted as a violation of group norms.[2] Dr. Vincent's disagreement with this partner, however, transcended both personal feelings and group norms. He claimed to have a different conception of the calling to medicine:

You know, we're really privy to information that no one else in the whole world is privy to, and because you are, it seems to me that it creates at least a responsibility on your part, first of all, to honor that, because it's got to be carried with a great amount of respect and privacy. [The youngest partner] always got angry with me because he said that I was a bleeding heart. But I think that sometimes you have to be overwhelmed by things you're told, and be overwhelmed by some of the unbelievable life experiences that people have.

He interpreted his conflict with his partner as indicative of a changing attitude among physicians about their responsibilities to patients. The accusation of "bleeding heart" was taken as an attack on his judgment, but he also construed it as evidence of his colleague's narrow ethic of care. In a world of diminishing expectations about the altruism of doctors, this minimalist ethic stood for much that Dr. Vincent disliked about his colleague and his profession.

He then told me a long story about his son, who had lost three fingers in an accident while moving logs. The boy was taken to a hospital an hour from Daleton where a special team of doctors attempted reattachment surgery. Dr. Vincent's inability to help his son was compounded by the behavior of the primary surgeon who performed the surgery:

> I was crying, and he talked to me about the Symphony Orchestra and some card players, friends that he plays with up here [in Daleton], while he was fiddling with our son's fingers that were in ice. We waited eighteen hours while he was in surgery, and they never came to talk to us, refused to take any of our calls. I didn't know what was going on at all. When it was over, they reattached his fingers and then they died. The fingers just didn't take and never would have taken, realistically . . . and I'm almost convinced that they did the surgery because I was a physician. . . . By the time the experience was over, my wife and I were so enraged at physicians in general because there was just so much a lack of humanity to us. And it just seemed to me that if I'm a physician and I were treated this way— there was not as much sensitivity as you'd give to a desk—I mean it was incredible! I still have a lot of anger directed towards the primary surgeon, just because he was such a bastard.

His emotional rage was directed against the pretense of medical concern rather than its real absence. The demand for "sensitivity" had little to do with the boy's treatment (which was excellent) and much to do with the treatment of the parents who anxiously awaited the outcome of surgery. Like the youngest partner in his former group, the primary surgeon in charge of his son took it for granted that providing excellent medical treatment to patients fulfilled his professional obligations; communication with anyone else about a patient's condition was not ethically demanded but was merely a matter of courtesy.

The experience of being on the other side of the physician-patient relation had a profound effect on Dr. Vincent's thinking about the calling to medicine:

There is this concept of an eight-to-four shift which more and more physicians are getting into. It seems that as a result, there's a loss of the humanism that must exist in medicine, recognizing that there's so much that we really don't know. Much of what we deal with in our field isn't life and death. Birth sometimes is, and cancer certainly is. But a lot of it are very painful and very emotionally exciting and traumatic events in life. I guess this past year [with his son's injury], I think it was probably part of what really forced me into the situation [of leaving the group], because my one partner just had no feelings and has no feelings. He will not deal with emotions at all. During the time that we were going through all this, he never once asked me how our child was. I think my wife and I just kind of came to the end point at the lack of sensitivity that existed towards us, that it really made us reevaluate our own approach to people.

His strong feelings about his partner were no longer expressed in the hope that the group would change; instead his partner's behavior came to symbolize what could not be changed, except by moving out on his own:

It seems to me you do need to remove yourself one step. You need to do that for your own sanity at times. But I think that you can so completely do that, that you remove from yourself the ability to feel pain or to feel sadness, or to feel happiness, or even sometimes just to admit that you can't cure somebody, or that somebody is going to die. . . . I have a little woman who is eighty-eight who has growing cancer of the cervix. And she's going to die. There's nothing that can be done about it. But the oncologist wanted to keep giving her chemotherapy and radiation therapy. She and I talked about it and decided that she wanted to die the way she is, and she didn't want anything else done to her. You know, you can do so much. You can do anything. There has to come a point in which you say, "My God! Would I do this to me or to my wife or to somebody that I really loved?" And if you can't say that, you have no right doing it. That's all been going on this past year. . . . In my own practice it got to the point where with [the youngest partner] I couldn't handle his inability to deal with the emotions. A large part of what I do is really that. There are bad diseases, but a lot of things are influenced by culture and environment, and by social circumstances, that really have nothing to do with medicine at all.

Dr. Vincent's move to solo practice was one of resignation as much as hope. The security of his occupation was never threatened, but his sense of vocation was redefined. His conversion to solo practice, then, marked a new resolve to do alone what could not be done better with colleagues. He remarked that many of the medical people he knew in Daleton were not supportive of his decision to leave group three, "because they feel that groups, at least in this community, separate only when people fight."

One of Dr. Vincent's partners, Dr. Hill, confirmed his claim that "there wasn't any kind of an internal squabble" that led to the breakup. Despite this denial, the subdividing of medical practices in Daleton was usually the outcome of personal rivalries and the desire to gain greater financial control over a practice, as in the case of Dr. Ingram and Dr. Simpson, described in chapter 3. One could argue that Dr. Vincent's move finally made economic sense and that, given his present ability to make it alone, personal differences in practice style now exceeded what he was willing to tolerate. The impetus to move might have expressed itself earlier if he had estimated that operating alone was economically feasible as well as beneficial to his family life. Yet the wish to begin a solo practice was by no means common to all physicians practicing in groups. Dr. Vincent's decision was a consequence of unexpected experiences that shook his confidence about how best to practice medicine.

Dr. Hill's opinion of his partner's decision to move into solo practice was quietly skeptical. He also emphasized the importance of free time and of family commitments by comparing their respective situations:

> I would never do it, because I do have family responsibilities and I can't be tied to the hospital a hundred percent of the time. He has one hundred percent responsibility for one hundred percent of his patients, a hundred percent of his time. My wife and family don't give me that permission. His wife and family gave him that permission. Even if you're not doing anything, you must be available, because that's what this kind of practice demands. There are things that I do with my family that take me out of state, and I can't practice that way. But I can't say that it's foolhardy, because he was obviously not being fulfilled as a person and as a physician in a group practice. He's a good doctor. He's very personable and tries to make himself available at all times. There will be just so many people he'll eventually be able to take care of, but he's going to be as busy as hell. He'll be as busy as he wants to be.

According to Dr. Hill, family and patients made special claims on a physician's work whether doctoring was done alone or in a group. One's stage of career also determined to a large extent when the opportunity to change practice would be financially realistic. But the desire to be "fulfilled as a person and as a physician" had an impact independent of these other constraints on medical practice.

Dr. Vincent's reservations about group practice developed from his particular conception of the calling of medicine. Dr. Hill's reservations about solo practice, especially in obstetrics, arose from the belief that group practice produced more efficient and reliable patient care; he also preferred the greater control over his own time that group practice afforded him. Yet, when he was on call, Dr. Hill disavowed the expediency, if not the virtue, of practicing in a group: "I always lose at tennis when I wear my beeper. . . . I never drink when I'm on call. There's nothing like a doctor coming to see a patient with booze on his breath." Aware that someone's life could depend on his physical and mental condition, Dr. Hill abstained from alcohol whenever it was his turn to answer calls from the hospital. When he was out of state with his family, he no longer considered himself on call. But at work for his group practice, he preserved the inner qualities of his calling to medicine. Solo practice would have demanded that he abstain continuously from alcohol because, in effect, he would have been always on call.[3]

The sense of obligation that both Dr. Vincent and Dr. Hill had to family and patients suggests that the altruism of medical work is deeply rooted in the melding of private and public time (Zerubavel, 1981:138–166). Both doctors agreed that group practice helped to maintain the separation between these two types of time, but Dr. Vincent was disappointed that this benefit had become more a right than a privilege: "I think sometimes you forget that it's really more than just a nine to five job. [The youngest partner] went off at five o'clock come hell or high water, and he didn't allow patients to ever get in his way. That always bothered me, and I couldn't deal with that." At this stage in his career, Dr. Vincent had decided that his public time in medicine was no less important than his private time. Separating family life from daily work has become a standard feature of modern life. The physician's calling tends to resist this separation between private and public by creating the expectation of what Eviatar

Zerubavel has called "ever-availability" (1981:146). In Dr. Vincent's case, the balancing of ever-availability with the demands of family changed over time.

Numerous characterizations have been made of medicine's corporate-style management of health, its organized insensitivity to the needs of patients, and its restraint of trade (see Freidson, 1970; Strauss, 1973; and Illich, 1976). Dr. Vincent believed that such criticisms fostered an image of doctoring that was powerful but one that diminished the patient's trust in the doctor. The charge against the conspiracy of professionals, of which a group practice was one possible manifestation, had profound effects on the specific interactions between physicians and patients. At the same time, the way in which physicians organized themselves—in order to reduce the demands made on them—was characteristic of many types of work in modern society. A patient's expectation that a physician's calling symbolized a constant, uninterrupted commitment to the practice of medicine was in large part illusory. Expectations, however, define situations, and a patient's trust depended greatly on the doctor's manner; a good doctor was more than technically good (see Apfel and Fisher, 1984:85ff.).

An unlisted telephone number was evidence of a physician's wish to maintain a separation between professional and private life. More than half Daleton's obstetrician/gynecologists had unlisted numbers. All but one doctor in solo practice listed their home numbers, while most in group practices did not. Dr. Vincent listed his number; Dr. Hill did not.[4] The growth of strategic forms of inaccessibility had many sources and manifestations. Specialization was certainly one source for the increased complexity of medicine and the use of referrals. In turn, the more transient quality of physician-patient relations, created by group practice, contributed to the separation of the lives of physicians and patients.

Dr. Vincent was convinced that more physicians than ever before practiced like Dr. Hill and the youngest partner in group three; their sense of vocation was demanding but was formed on their own terms. He complained that the practice of medicine had been subordinated to the interests of group efficiency and cost-effectiveness. His idealistic move into solo practice was intended to reestablish a personal presence and trust that would resist the seemingly inevitable movement toward a more encompassing management of medical work by business and government.

The complex nature of trust and sensitivity was further revealed in Dr. Vincent's remarks about his marriage. Chapter 4 reports his wife's initial reactions to his changed view of abortion: she was disturbed by the fact that he could believe in a woman's "right" to elect the procedure but was no longer willing to perform it. He conceded that when he had tried to understand his wife's emotions about a miscarriage she suffered early in their marriage, it was as difficult for him to do so as he imagined it must have been for her to understand his position on abortion:

> We lost a pregnancy about twelve weeks, and I can remember I was a medical intern, and I can remember my wife aborting in the toilet. It was a little glob, you know. And at that time, I can remember saying, "Well, gee, honey. You're not having any problems." She didn't have to go to the hospital. I can remember that she was really devastated. I didn't remember feeling anything and I didn't at that point in my life really understand what her feelings were, and why she was so bothered by it. I was ignorant and not able to respond to my own wife's needs at that time. I didn't understand it, and dealing with it all the time now, I've kept an ear out for what happens after those experiences. To have physicians say, "Well, there'll be another pregnancy" is really kind of hollow advice.

Dr. Vincent's growth as a physician was rooted in the practice rather than the knowledge of medicine. Inspired at first by the medical knowledge of probabilities, he did not understand his wife's dilemma. Her case became the prototype for his future responses to patients. Medical learning alone does not guarantee that a physician will develop what Thomas McKeown has called a "pastoral" role (1979:134–135). "Hollow advice" was initially all Dr. Vincent could offer.

Trust in the physician is a function of expertise, but it is also established in the assurances that are made between people, not only between test results and patients (see McDermott, 1981:840). The pastoral role in medicine is perhaps diminished because it does not lend itself easily to being formulated as knowledge. With the enormous literature on ethics produced largely outside of, but about, the profession, new expectations about the practice of medicine have arisen. The doctor's sense of responsibility has become more complex, if only as a function of the greater knowledge that has been produced about it.

Daleton physicians were generally unfamiliar with the literature on bioethics and the attempts of ethicists to work in partnership with doctors to improve the quality of medical care. The moral to be drawn from the reactions of Dr. Vincent and Dr. Hill is that inner direction persists in the physician's character despite movements to organize this character in other-directed ways. In this sense, many efforts to introduce ethics into medical and clinical curricula have unwittingly conformed with the specialized, fragmented image of medicine, if only because ethics becomes one more form of knowledge that requires experts to impart to those less able to discern how medicine should be practiced.

Innovation beyond Private Practice

The relative confidence of Daleton practitioners in the practice of medicine was circumscribed by uncertainties that have little to do with physician character or the specific social relations among colleagues.[5] For example, during the past decade, the use of amniocentesis to determine the health (and incidentally the sex) of the unborn has taken on increased importance in the practice of medicine (see Rosenstock et al., 1975; Capron et al., 1979; and President's Commission for the Study of Ethical Problems in Medicine and Biomedical and Behavioral Research, 1983). The development of techniques to detect and classify a variety of genetic anomalies that might result in the birth of deformed or ill infants has created a new responsibility for doctors to offer amniocentesis to their patients.

Physicians in Daleton indicated that they routinely recommended the procedure to women over thirty-five, at which age the probability of giving birth to a child with Down syndrome significantly increases. For the patient and her family, amniocentesis is intended to reassure them that a particular pregnancy will end in the birth of a genetically normal child. On the rare occasion when abnormalities are detected, the woman must decide whether to undergo an abortion, usually between the fifteenth and eighteenth weeks of pregnancy.

For the physician, amniocentesis poses a risk to the health of the mother and her unborn child. The withdrawal of amniotic fluid from the mother's amniotic sac requires practice and adeptness. Several physicians explained that they carefully maintained records of their offer (and their view of the risks) in case they were later sued for malpractice. They had to be legally prepared to defend their actions if the amniocentesis injured the mother or her unborn child or if a negative diagnosis (that is, the determination that no genetic defects were evident) proved upon birth to be incorrect. Patients were also informed of the possibility of a false positive diagnosis. The innovation was cautiously assessed in light of these medical uncertainties and legal complications.

The keeping of meticulous medical records became a strategy to avoid these complications, but it was by no means foolproof. One doctor said that he practiced "defensive" medicine, which included describing all the possible risks associated with different procedures as well as ordering an extensive (and expensive) battery of tests:

> Defensive medicine is the routine in our specialty. If a lawyer for the plaintiff were to come up with one scientific report about the risks associated with any treatment I had given, say, for ovarian cancer, I would tell my lawyer to find a study which said the treatment was the best available. The threat of malpractice is terrible for the doctor who may know that there are two conflicting reports about the same treatment. But if the scientists disagree, what can be expected of doctors?

In Daleton, medical treatments were intended to be therapeutic rather than experimental. The risks associated with using them were calculated in terms of the physician's own knowledge and ability. Mistakes in routine diagnosis, for instance, would be blamed on the doctor. But this was not the case for amniocentesis. In fact, although the procedure was performed in Daleton, the amniotic fluid was sent outside the community for analysis. Waiting for word from other experts, physicians knew they would have to act on the results of major tests over which they had little control.

Accustomed to seeing the short-term advantages or disadvantages of a specific course of treatment, doctors charted that course on the basis of the patient's response and the best available medical knowledge of what should be done. As with abortion, the development of treatments that were not intended primarily to cure disease created new uncertainties about the levels of acceptable risk to the patient and the physician.

With the availability of genetic screening, tremendous pressure has

asserted itself, especially among the middle and upper classes, to produce genetically normal infants. The potential risk to the unborn is
now seen as an opportunity: it is tragic, some say, to act against a
normal fetus as the result of a false positive diagnosis, but it is more
tragic not to diagnose an abnormal one. Physicians in Daleton accepted the procedure in principle as statistically safe. They also were
aware that injuries to mothers and normal fetuses could occasionally
occur but were unanimous about their responsibilities for counseling
patients.[6] The medical risks to patients were balanced against the
legal liabilities to their medical practices. Even Catholic physicians
opposed to abortion admitted that it was occasionally in their own
best interests to inform patients of the availability of the procedure
and refer them to someone who would perform it. Daleton's Catholic
doctors who refused to perform abortions also did not perform amniocentesis.

The number of requests for amniocentesis in Daleton was not large.
Several physicians said that they had performed the procedure, but
no physician said that he had ever been faced with a positive diagnosis.
Amniocentesis was readily available outside the community, where
genetic counseling services were more extensively developed. In
Daleton obstetrician/gynecologists doubled as genetic counselors. The
use of referral for second-trimester abortions was especially evident
in the case of amniocentesis. Referral protected physicians against
charges of legal negligence and technical incompetence. The legal
and medical complications of amniocentesis did not deter them from
acting on behalf of patients, but they were careful to outline all the
possible exceptions to the statistical rules. The new expectation that
they would be responsible for determining whether infants would
be born genetically normal demanded that they acknowledge their
role in the technological advances of their profession. From the
standpoint of private practice, these advances could be adopted or
observed from a distance.

Unlike amniocentesis, the contraceptive pill was an innovation
adopted by every physician in the community, though circumstances
for its prescription varied. In 1981 alone, more than fifty-five million
prescriptions for the pill were written by doctors throughout the
country (see *Journal of the American Medical Association,* 1984).[7] Be-

cause of its widespread use, the pill has been subject to increased scrutiny by epidemiologists who have attempted to estimate its short- and long-term effects on health. The focus on the probabilities of harm from using the pill has also led to studies of the benefits and risks of other forms of birth control, such as the cervical cap and Depo-Provera.

One physician in the community had been authorized to prescribe a newly designed cervical cap by the pharmaceutical company that manufactured it. He had notified federal authorities of his intention to prescribe it provisionally and had informed patients that the results of their use of the cap would be reported to the drug company, which in turn would submit its collective findings to the federal government. This bureaucratically conducted experiment in an innovative form of birth control would, the physician predicted, take many years.

Physicians in Daleton had heard of Depo-Provera, but none had ever worked with it. The drug is capable of suppressing ovulation for three months or longer with a single injection. One physician was aware that it was available outside the United States and compared its use in the Third World to his use of the IUD here. The morbidity and mortality associated with such forms of birth control, he maintained, had to be weighed against the benefits of controlling population (see Sun, 1982).

The uncertainties that physicians faced with the pill were exemplified by the "informational insert" (that is, brochure) supplied with each prescription. Dr. Evans of group six prescribed the pill to younger patients who requested birth control and to older, post-menopausal, patients for whom estrogen was sometimes indicated. He discussed how he handled questions about the various warnings contained in the insert:

> I know I spend at least an hour a day, if not two, talking about that estrogen insert that the Government puts in this product. It's the biggest pain in the rear-end that they ever thought of! Many, many patients who desperately need to take estrogen just will not take it. Now a woman whose vagina got so dry and so tight that she just no longer has intercourse—and she just tells her husband to drop dead, to buzz off and the marriage is disrupted, everything, because she's not willing to use a little estrogen. There isn't any way in this world that that's going to be harmful to her. Usually these are women who have had hysterectomies and they

don't even have a uterus to get cancer in, but they're just so uptight and neurotic about the thing that they won't use estrogen. Now I can talk myself blue in the face, but who are you? You're just a doctor. You don't know anything about it.

Dr. Evans' authority as a doctor was challenged by the uncertain nature of the substance he prescribed. A patient could easily see from reading the insert that the physician was no better informed than anyone else about the long-term effects of taking the pill. After consulting with a physician about its possible side effects, the patient would learn that neither the manufacturer nor her doctor could guarantee that there would be no long-term health risks from using the pill. A patient's informed consent meant only that she was aware of the medical uncertainties of taking the pill.

From Dr. Evans' point of view, candor about medical risks had become a matter of common sense in the face of potentially litigious patients:

> I think it's good for patients to be well informed and make their own decisions. In a way, it makes it easier for me because I don't feel liable for the decision. I try to educate them as best as I can to the pros and cons, and let them make their own decision. I'll say, "Now you go home and here's a prescription. If you want it, you fill it, and if you don't want it, forget it. It's your decision. I can teach you about it but I can't decide what you should do." And I'll find myself escaping from the liability and the anxiety just simply by approaching it this way. And even in the case of surgery, I rarely say, "You must have this operation."

The nonjudgmental approach to doctoring happened to coincide with the development of treatments that fell somewhere on a continuum between medically necessary and patient-elected. Like first-trimester abortions and amniocentesis, the pill was more often prescribed because it was asked for than because it was medically necessary. By giving patients a series of options, Dr. Evans was able to escape from "liability and anxiety." He also acknowledged the diminished nature of his authority to act on their behalf.

At the same time, the notion of "long-term" risk was antithetical to Dr. Evans' practice of medicine. He described circumstances that had an immediate impact on patients' lives, such as the possible breakup of a marriage because of the wife's inability to participate in intercourse, and he compared these circumstances to a patient's anxiety about potential future risks to health from using the pill. His nonjudgmental stance was a pretense of sorts, behind which he criticized patients' uncertainties about the dangers of treatment:

> This estrogen insert—they don't put things in perspective. Every other word in that thing is "cancer" and they make you think that if you take the pill, you're going to drop dead the next minute. I don't refute anything that's in there. Some of it is debatable, but if it even might be true, it's worthwhile taking that into consideration when you decide about the medicine. Even if it is true, it's just so unlikely or rare or seldom that those things occur, and you have about a hundred percent chance of your marriage busting up when you tell the old man to get lost, whereas you might have one chance in a billion of getting some weird hepatic carcinoma because you've taken estrogen. . . .
>
> There's another insert they give with progesterone which says it can cause birth defects. If that's true at all, it's just a very small fraction of a percent, and you've got a 6 percent chance of having a birth defect across the board—if you take progesterone, maybe it goes from 6 to 6.1 percent. Well, it's such a miniscule amount that it doesn't make any sense in a practical way. Now when they understand this, they think, "Well, you're right, Doctor. It's silly."

Dr. Evans' patients were supposed to be reassured by probabilities. But he realized that the uncertainties inherent in probabilities were responsible in part for patients' growing distrust of medical expertise:

> If a woman basically is a trusting type of person that you've had a good relationship with, she'll believe you. You can work with her. But there are a whole lot of people that are so suspicious of doctors and the medical profession that there is absolutely nothing that you can say. I just say, "Well, let's not waste your time and mine. I know where you're coming from; there's nothing I'll ever say that will change your mind."

The "trusting type of person" could be dissuaded from believing that all the possible risks applied specifically to her. Dr. Evans admitted that he could do nothing about those who would not listen. His expertise was compromised in the assumption that he was wasting his time in trying to change their minds.

Dr. Evans' commitment to patients shifted between what P. M. Strong has described as the "bureaucratic format" and the "charity format" (1983:67–68; see also Strong, 1979). On the one hand,

Dr. Evans spoke of "options" as if the patient were perfectly competent to distinguish among them. On the other hand, he stressed his firm belief in the scientific efficacy of certain treatments and chastised patients, at least indirectly, for their unwillingness to accept his clinical judgment. The bureaucratic format protected his professional autonomy, but his calling to medicine was also expressed in his adamant conviction that he sometimes knew what was best for patients.

A patient's distrust of medical expertise was the result of uncertainty and something more substantial, as Dr. Evans observed:

> I think doctors over the last twenty years have through health insurances become so well established that they've seen this as a windfall and have taken advantage of the situation to their own financial benefit. In the process of doing this, they've lost touch with the people that they originally had more concern about. I think materialism has all but wrecked the medical profession. It isn't a ministry any more, it's not a dedication. It's a business. It's a way of making a lot of money in a hurry, and retiring or continuing so you have all the more to spend. When I went into medicine it was like a minister, or a rabbi, or a priest. You devoted your life to these people and if you got rich or you didn't get rich, it didn't matter. What mattered was the way you served your people. You don't see doctors like that.

The changes in the practice of medicine were reflected in physician character as much as in the innovations of medical practice and treatments. Like Dr. Vincent, Dr. Evans directed criticisms against certain changes in modern medical practice, but both men also lamented a change in the calling itself.

The Fate of Idealism in Private Practice

Over twenty-five years ago, Howard S. Becker and Blanche Geer concluded in "The Fate of Idealism in Medical School" that although medical students tended to develop cynical feelings about medicine in specific situations associated with their medical school experience, they never lost their original idealism about the profession, their belief that "medicine is a wonderful thing" and that once they became physicians they would "devote their lives to service to mankind" (1958:50–51). Concern about abortion figured in this view:

Their original idealism reasserts itself as the end of school approaches. Seniors show more interest than students in earlier years in serious ethical dilemmas of the kind they expect to face in practice. They have become aware of ethical problems laymen often see as crucial for the physician—whether it is right to keep patients with fatal diseases alive as long as possible, or what should be done if an influential patient demands an abortion—and worry about them. (p. 54)

Becker and Geer proposed that a new professional idealism emerged at the end of medical school that confined the physician's calling more specifically to the welfare of patients. The physician was expected always to examine patients thoroughly and "to give treatment based on firm diagnosis rather than merely to relieve symptoms" (p. 55).

In various ways, abortion, amniocentesis, and the pill challenged the physician's professional responsibility "to give treatment based on firm diagnosis rather than merely to relieve symptoms." Having the legal responsibility for performing abortions did not enlighten physicians with regard to their medical duties. On the contrary, many of them had difficulty reconciling their personal wish to help patients with their feelings about the medical status of abortion. Was abortion a medical treatment or simply a procedure that a licensed physician was required to perform? Was the pill a medical treatment or simply a substance that a licensed physician was required to prescribe? The unanimous professional acceptance of amniocentesis was due to its clearly diagnostic character: but was an abortion following a positive diagnosis a medical treatment or merely a way to relieve symptoms?

Whether or not innovations in diagnosis and treatment were adopted depended on a physician's definition of the medical situation. Controversial innovations were to a large extent on the professional fringes of medical practice in Daleton. Physicians' acceptance of first-trimester abortion was comparable to their acceptance of most forms of medical and surgical treatment for infertility. Yet, as in the case of second-trimester abortion, treatment for infertility was questioned more carefully when physicians discussed the technical development of in vitro fertilization. At the frontier of the scientifically monitored creation of human life, the matter of abortion reappeared, especially in connection with the disposal of fertilized eggs that were not implanted in the uterus (see Walters and Singer, 1982, and Arditti *et al.*, 1984).

The few places in the United States offering in vitro fertilization stood in the same relationship to the community of Daleton as did the clinics to which many patients were referred for abortions. By maintaining a split between the routines of their medical practices and the innovations in technique and treatment occurring in clinics and laboratories outside Daleton, local practitioners were able to resolve many of their uncertainties about their professional responsibilities. The attempt by Dr. Evans and others to introduce new birthing innovations in the community challenged the way some physicians participated in the control of events. This challenge to practice style, however, did not compare to other innovations that imposed medically and legally problematic expectations on physicians. Private practice was a refuge from the pressures to conform to innovations of any kind. In one sense, the practice of medicine in Daleton represented the lag between innovation and adoption. In another sense, individual physicians in private practice were able to decide how quickly and to what degree the process of adoption would occur.

The fate of idealism among physicians in private practice was determined in two ways. On the one hand, Daleton doctors were able to control the conditions of their medical practices by using referrals, by specializing in some techniques and not in others, and by choosing to practice alone or in a group. Upon completion of residency, the normative constraints, so powerful a part of medical training until then, were abruptly diffused. The younger practitioners remained "test-wise" in anticipation of board certification, but other than this symbolic reminder of their connection to the larger profession, physicians in private practice no longer experienced the constant awareness of being scrutinized by superordinates.

On the other hand, the fate of idealism in private practice was determined by circumstances that were often beyond the control of any individual practitioner. Historian of science Barbara Gutmann Rosenkrantz has observed:

> Although the relationships between physicians and patients are highly personal, the basis for mutual understanding has been fundamentally altered in this century by shared confidence in science. Despite warnings

that science cannot produce miracles, the disruptive consequences of disease have been reordered primarily by scientifically authorized medical institutions and practices. Personal and social experiences that define and determine health and disease have changed because of the expectation that the relationship of cause and effect discerned in nature permits scientific medical interventions. Physicians and patients have continued to acknowledge that mediating personal exchanges shape their encounters with each other and with the intrusive agents of disease, but at the same time they have come to depend on science to mitigate and justify the differences that separate them. (1979:5)[8]

The formulation of risk in medical treatment has become inseparable from the expectation that the effects of treatment can be determined for every individual under every circumstance. For Daleton doctors, a human life itself was the long measure between cause and effect. Like the demand for equal well-being, the achievement of universal criteria for medical treatment stood beyond the reality of human differences that no degree of control, political or medical, could completely overcome. Private practice acted as a barrier between a profession that ideally served humanity and the physician who first served individual patients.

7
Beyond
the Politics
of Abortion

In their study of *Middletown Families: Fifty Years of Change and Continuity*, conducted between 1976 and 1981, Theodore Caplow *et al.* reported that in the "telephone company's yellow pages for 1978, the first entry was abortion information, followed by the instruction 'See birth control information centers.'" Twelve centers were listed, eleven of which "explicitly advertised abortion services. The exception was Middletown's own Planned Parenthood clinic" (1982:183). Like Middletown, Daleton did not have an abortion clinic, and the Daleton yellow pages also listed the names of such clinics, all of which were outside the community.

In another study, published in *Family Planning Perspectives* in 1980, Sara Seims concluded that "in eight out of 10 U.S. counties, containing more than one-quarter of U.S. women estimated to be in need of abortion services in 1977, no physician, clinic or hospital provided abortions." Seims pointed out that although some counties did have providers of abortion services, this did not guarantee that women would be able to obtain them. "In many instances, this is because the abortion providers consist of private physicians who perform abortions for their own patients in their offices or in hospitals, but who do not serve women whom they do not know (1980:88; see also Forrest *et al.*, 1979a, and Robinson, 1979).

The sociological significance of abortion availability in the United States has yet to be fully assessed in light of the fact that private practice continues to serve as the major barrier to a more equitable provision of this procedure. Both independence and inconsistency defined this practice among obstetrician/gynecologists in Daleton. My effort to understand their medical practices centered first on how they negotiated requests for abortion. The majority supported the right of physicians to determine when a pregnancy should be interrupted; the question of the patient's right to make the same decision was faced more theoretically. Referral became the practical response to the general problem of patients' rights.

The practice of obstetrics and gynecology was split apart at many levels of its organization. Subspecialization enabled some doctors to avoid ever being faced with the decision to perform an abortion. Others elected not to do obstetrics. Physicians in group practices organized themselves so that each member could determine what he would and would not do. The division between obstetrics and gynecology was expressed as much in the social organization of abortion services as in many doctors' wishes to prevent gynecology from becoming obstetrics. In their nearly unanimous avoidance of second-trimester abortions, Daleton doctors acknowledged the differences between birth and birth control.

Each practitioner in Daleton was guided by a strong sense of self-preservation. Each was reluctant to become too deeply involved with the personal lives of patients or with the political aims of social movements for and against abortion. Their reactions to questions about the Hippocratic oath were indicative of this professional aversion to controversial aspects of their work.

When asked how they reconciled the liberalizing of abortion with Hippocrates' injunction against it ("I will not give a woman a pessary to cause abortion"), they referred to the oath as "small potatoes," "never to be taken literally," "a nicety," "not binding," "an anachronism," "a pleasant custom," and "meaningless." Several explained that the oath's prohibition of abortion was an expression of concern about the dangers of primitive technology. One observed that in Hippocrates' time, abortion "was bad news for everybody," while another remarked that "in those days there was an 80 percent mortality rate for induced abortions."

Others thought that the entire oath was open to interpretation.

One claimed that "the Oath is so old that in time it has deteriorated a little. You must establish your own ethics." Another pointed out that there were many interpretations of the Bible and the Ten Commandments. "I have recited the Ten Commandments a couple of times too, and I probably broke a couple." He said that he had never given a pessary to produce abortion, although he had performed many abortions. A Catholic practitioner on staff at St. Timothy indicated that he took the injunction against abortion literally but conceded, "You've got to qualify it [the injunction] today. It doesn't hold one hundred percent. In our own church we have concepts which wouldn't have been accepted ten years ago." Finally, one younger doctor admitted, "You can't believe everything you say. We all say lies."

Dr. Simpson of group one thought that the oath had outlived its usefulness: "It should be updated, rewritten. The Vatican has already applied the same principle. Now it's OK to eat meat on Friday."

All but three physicians in Daleton remembered taking the oath. One had not attended his graduation, and two could not remember whether they had actually taken it. Several had sworn to an abbreviated version in which the entire passage on abortion had been deleted. One recounted: "Students were told they did not have to repeat any part of the Oath which they did not believe. I didn't study it in great detail. But now that I think about it, it's interesting. Maybe I'll have to change my view." Ancient stipulations about the practice of medicine were translated into modern responses to the demands of medical practice. Those demands appeared to place abortion, and family planning generally, on the fringes of medical practice.

If obstetrician/gynecologists living in Daleton had read the local newspaper during the late 1970s and early 1980s, they would have been made aware of the fact that their commitment to medical practice over and against the politics of abortion did not necessarily protect them from public controversy. For example, an Associated Press news story on April 11, 1978, reported the shooting of an Italian gynecologist:

> Monday night, three men and two women raided the office of a Turin gynecologist, Ruggero Grio, and shot him in the legs and shoulders. The raiders apparently were from the Armed Proletarian Squads, a small ultra-leftist group that is not known to have any connection with the Red

Brigades. It was believed that they blamed Grio for the death of a woman who died of an illegal abortion after he refused to operate on her.

A United Press International report on June 7, 1978, displayed the following headline: Doctors Are Warned in Italy. The first paragraph of the report stated:

> The Roman Catholic Vicar of Rome warned Tuesday that any Catholic doctor performing an abortion under Italy's new law would be excommunicated from the Church.

The events in Italy at that time were far removed from the private practices of physicians in Daleton. But reports about the firebombing of abortion clinics in this country and the kidnapping of clinic supervisors confirmed the real politics of abortion that Daleton physicians actively and effectively avoided.

The medical profession has been subject to considerable hostility because it remains the sole legal provider of abortion. Its authority over this procedure could be disestablished in at least two ways: nonphysicians could be authorized to perform abortions, or physicians could be compelled to perform them whenever a patient requests one. Neither course is likely to be acceptable to medical professionals, the courts, or, for that matter, the operators of the established system of abortion clinics in this country.

A third way exists that could diffuse the profession's authority over abortion. The prospects for a do-it-yourself home abortion kit have been sounded from time to time. Physicians in Daleton were generally opposed to this development because they claimed that any method of aborting a pregnancy poses risks. They were also reluctant to give paramedical personnel surgical responsibilities. One physician said: "There are an awful lot of physicians I would not like to have doing suction curettage. The first-trimester abortion is a technically simple procedure but there should always be medical back-up available." Another was adamantly opposed to legislation that would allow anyone who was not medically licensed to perform abortions: "If the government steps into medicine, I'll put down my scepter and pick up a sword. They [abortions] have to be done right. It is a mistake not to have surgically qualified people who have had other surgical experience when doing these procedures." Several other doctors were less anxious about the medical risks. One proposed that nonphysician personnel could become more important if the demand for abortion were to increase significantly. He maintained that first-trimester abortions "are very easy to do. Nurses could do them."

Physicians agreed less on who should perform abortions than on how they should be performed. The moral imperative to perform them technically well gave no guidance as to when they should be performed. In this way, private practice was both a source of and protection from the politics of abortion.

The physician today is nearly invisible in the American controversy over abortion. This is due in part to the fact that a relatively small number of physicians perform the vast majority of abortions. In an important study of obstetrician/gynecologists' rationales for accepting and refusing requests for abortion, Constance A. Nathanson and Marshall H. Becker concluded: "A major consequence of obstetrical conservatism in the United States has been that women have had limited access to abortion within the traditional health care system; currently, the large majority of abortions take place outside the system in private, single-purpose abortion clinics" (1981:209). Until the legalization of abortion, family planning evoked little public controversy. The objectives of family planners were middle-class hopes of producing the optimal-size family along with appropriately spaced children. With abortion came the mobilization of social movements that split the alliance between family and planning. Obstetrical conservatism was one outcome of this ideological transformation of family planning out of which developed two distinctive forms of medical work: obstetrical and nonobstetrical family planning. Physicians' control over obstetrical work was challenged but not fundamentally changed. Their control over abortion, however, reflected a legal mandate with no corresponding professional consensus about when the procedure was medically indicated. In one sense, the abortion clinic became the organizational response to professional ambivalence about the place of abortion in medical practice.

The social control of medical expertise has historically been accomplished by physicians themselves. The fact that they are of many different minds about their obligations to patients with respect to abortion and birth control points to a lack of conscious professional attempts to control their work in these matters. Of course, epidemiological knowledge has proved to be an effective agent of control over the types of methods used to accomplish abortion. But within the profession itself, not even the standardization of technical care for first-trimester abortion has resulted in an equitable delivery of this service by physicians.

For the physician in practice in Daleton, the pro-life attempts to dictate when abortions should not be performed were functionally similar to the pro-choice attempts to determine when they should be performed. Between competing pressures to organize how medicine should be practiced, each physician reserved the right to decide how it would be practiced. Private practice preserved a space in which to work despite such pressures. Professional autonomy was a source of authority for the physician, but it also served as a means for escaping the publicly, if not technically, controversial aspects of medical work.

All physicians in Daleton indicated that if elective abortions were made illegal again, they would not perform them. It would appear that the legacy of illegal abortion still asserted itself in their responses to the prospect of a constitutional amendment giving states the right to determine when abortion could be performed. The bold autonomy of professionalism, the physician's right to decide, was given up without hesitation in the face of the law. Complications of a legal kind were feared most: the ever higher premiums on malpractice insurance are perhaps one of the few real social taxes for the privilege of professional autonomy.

As we have seen, the original impetus for state control of abortion came primarily from the medical profession in the second half of the nineteenth century. The entanglement of state and profession was undone to a large extent with the legalization of the procedure. But a haunting ambivalence persisted in the actions of physicians in private practice, who balanced legal freedom with medical necessity in different ways.

Because the women's movement has often been cited as a major social force challenging the state and professional monopoly over restrictive abortion law, it is important to ask whether abortion services in this country will be organized much differently in the future. Regardless of physicians' private reasons for referring abortion requests, their refusals to offer abortion services have had the same public consequences. By deflecting requests to other providers, practitioners have reinforced the market stronghold that the larger clinics maintain over abortion. Michael S. Goldstein has provided compelling evidence that the existing markets of mass-produced abortion services, besides being created by physician entrepreneurs, have been controlled primarily by men, who continue to perform the largest numbers of abortions (1984a, 1984b).[1] The expectation of any changes in the delivery of these services as the result of the increased numbers of women in medicine must be assessed with these facts in mind.

The freedom of women to choose abortion has been constrained by more than the market forces that have led to its present lopsided provision. The service rendered has been subject to moralization for so long that contemporary providers have been discredited by their professional peers. The change in law has exposed the moral underside of professional status, of which "abortionist" is the best-known example. To imagine that innovations in law and technique will necessarily produce changes in the moral sensibilities of an entire profession is sociologically and politically naive. Physicians were once the moral entrepreneurs *against* abortion. The existence of this moral legacy remains an important factor in the lack of accommodation of the practice of medicine to abortion.

From all reports, the ambiguous status of abortion in the American repertoire of birth control suggests that other cultural factors have contributed to the professional and social stigmatization of abortion. Among the most significant is the legacy of the American birth-control movement. That movement began outside and against medicine but later won over the profession, whose involvement increased significantly after the introduction of the pill in the 1960s. From this movement originated the contemporary notion of the right to birth control. As one of their major strategies, movement leaders asserted that the right to birth control did not extend to abortion; in fact, abortion was consistently depicted as inferior, technically and morally.

The improvement of the technical safety of abortion demolished one part of this strategy; the other part continues to influence how contemporary observers reason about the different methods of birth control available. Historian James Reed has written:

In the 1970s the pill and the IUD still had not made contraception stress or risk free, and interest remains high in the prospects for still better technology. Perhaps the hope for a new technological fix, the persistent desire to separate contraception from coitus, reflects a naive attitude toward sex, the need to avoid responsibility or to maintain some myth of spontaneity. No one ever died from using a condom. Nor do diaphragms cause excessive menstruation or pelvic infections. In a rational society fertility could be controlled without "physiological" contraception or sexual repression. Society's need for the pill and the IUD might then be regarded as symbols of our lack of sex education, a measure of the persistence of dysfunctional attitudes from the past. (1978:376)

Sociologist Kristin Luker has expressed similar concerns about the direction of social policy with respect to abortion:

This does not mean, however, that we are ready to argue that abortion should be popularized as one of several equally acceptable methods of fertility control, with the same techniques used to encourage women to get abortions as are now used to encourage them to use contraception. Although the actual delivery of abortion necessarily reflects its present status as a major method of fertility control, it is not clear that this necessarily means we should make an ideological commitment to it as a long-term method, or that we should abandon research into better contraceptives with lower social costs for both men and women. . . . What the social and technological spinoffs of abortion as a socially preferred method of fertility control are, we can only speculate. (1975:147)

Both Reed and Luker acknowledge that some form of moral valuation is implicit in the distinctions made about different methods of birth control. Especially among physicians, abortion has been technically but not morally routinized. The paradox of abortion for the profession is that, when performed by a competent physician during the first trimester of pregnancy, the procedure is technically one of the safest forms of birth control. The pill and the IUD have been associated with a far wider variety of complications.

Yet the performance of an abortion is also a social encounter in a way that the prescription of a pill or the insertion of a device is not. The ideology of safety and efficiency has not altered the social basis for the performance of abortion, and here, perhaps, is another reason why physicians *and* patients have implicitly agreed to accept the possibly higher risks of pharmaceutical contraception. Among relatively marginal groups of feminist health advocates, abortion has acquired a high degree of acceptance precisely because of its technical safety. In the absence of moral valuations about it (for example, as an inferior form of birth control), its use along with mechanical forms of birth control (for example, the condom and diaphragm) may produce the least morbidity among the largest number of women. This points to a profound conflict between modern rationality and the cultural legacies that have condemned abortion as an inferior form of birth control.

In her more recent thinking about the prospects for reducing the resort to abortion in America, Kristin Luker has grown less sanguine:

> My personal and professional experiences have convinced me of several inescapable conclusions. First, there is no reason to assume that the answer to the abortion problem is contraception. Americans smoke, drive when they've been drinking, and steadfastly refuse to fasten their seat belts. Why should we expect contraceptive behavior to be of a higher standard, when everyone agrees that correct behavior in these other areas can literally save lives? Unintended pregnancies, like lung cancer and automobile deaths, are a fact of life. The only real policy choice that confronts Americans is whether a significant portion of those pregnancies will be ended legally or illegally. . . . Finally, I am convinced that this policy choice cannot be made rationally. Feelings about abortion draw too much on deeply held, tacit values about the meaning of life for people to admit of any compromise. (1984a:26)

Given this assessment, the high hopes of an earlier day appear to be very dim. At one time, abortion and birth control were viewed as moral opposites; to advocate birth control meant to challenge the assertion that "unintended pregnancies are a fact of life." Contemporary despair about reducing the resort to abortion means that no one—not women, men, or physicians—can be held to a higher standard. But that standard persists, despite all generalizations against it, because abortion remains morally unroutinized, at least outside the culture of clinics.

Ambivalence and uncertainty about abortion should not be confused with legal-bureaucratic norms about how it should be made available. Those norms now permit its performance for any reason, but this does not mean that all physicians will perform abortions for any reason. Discouraging a particular action is not the moral equivalent of outlawing it. Why must the question of a social policy on abortion be abandoned simply because "feelings about abortion draw too much on deeply held, tacit values about the meaning of life"? Within the province of medicine, those values have produced a version of compromise that has led to the present delivery of abortion services in the United States. That it may be unsatisfactory to both sides of the political issue reflects an irrationality at the level of politics.

On the one hand, the belief exists that abortion can never be stopped and that therefore all attempts to reduce it are useless. On the other hand, the belief exists that no circumstance warrants abortion. Between these two beliefs, the approval and disapproval of abortion rests in the hands of those who request it and those who perform it. The question I pose for those in the right-to-life movement is whether abortion will in fact become unavailable if a law is passed against it (see Noonan, 1979). The question I pose for those in the right-to-choose movement is whether abortion will become unavailable if efforts are made to discourage it without resort to outlawing it again (see Jaffe *et al.*, 1981). Compromise between these movements might begin by their acceptance of the idea that abortion should remain legal while strong public efforts are made, as they are increasingly made with respect to drinking and smoking, to discourage it.[2] In this way, a social policy for abortion could treat the legal right seriously without having to approve of every individual case. The question for pro-choice forces is whether they will acknowledge that the practice of abortion is a legal right that can be moralized against. The question for pro-life forces is whether they will acknowledge that reducing the practice of abortion is a more rational aim than passing unenforceable laws.

Contemporary moralizing about abortion has, of course, focused mainly on the status of the unborn and the right of women to control reproduction. Physicians in Daleton were well aware of the public interpretations of their abortion work. In the context of medical practice, advances in obstetrical care paralleled improvements in abortion procedures. The monitoring of birth was a major technical preoccupation that intensified the differences between obstetrics and abortion. Yet physicians were no more likely to concede a right to life than a right to abortion. Their ambivalence was expressed in the organization of their medical practices. They emphasized their reputations, their professional certifications, and, most important, *their* right to determine their medical responsibilities.

Since Taussig's time, medical indications for abortion have all but disappeared. Those indications once justified a physician's participation, but they did not compel a woman to undergo abortion. The right to choose whether to perform an abortion has placed the physician in a position analogous to that of the patient who was told that an abortion was medically indicated. Now the physician is asked to decide on the basis of the reasons presented by the patient. If abortion were morally routinized like other forms of birth control, the physician's responsibility would be no more problematic than it is in the prescribing of the pill or the fitting of a diaphragm. The major difference is that physicians are required to participate in the accomplishment of abortion. The pill, in contrast, does not involve the physician so personally and directly. Unlike any other form of birth control, abortion disrupts the taken-for-granted meanings of privacy and sexuality.

The social organization of abortion services in the United States must be explained by more than strictly economic factors. Whatever deterred physicians in Daleton from performing large numbers of abortions was also part of the cultural legacy of the medical profession. As political forces in the larger society battle to determine whether abortion will remain legal, the profession of medicine has already expressed its reservations about rights on both sides of the issue. I am inclined to agree with historian James C. Mohr's argument that the prohibition against abortion was an aberration in American history, a brief interval between a time when its practice was ignored and when it was permitted with protection from the highest court in the land (1978:255–63). The medical profession once sought to use the law to bring about new standards in technical care. Abortion itself, since legalization, has been brought under those standards.

What remains to be seen is whether its moral routinization will also be accomplished. Because the public issue of abortion centers for some people on its accessibility and safety and for others on the inviolability of unborn life, the attempts to define contraceptive responsibility over and against abortion have lost much of their force to shape consensus between opposing sides. Rhetorics of sexual and contraceptive responsibility have been overshadowed by litigiously inspired defenses of individual right, as if there were no other systems of protection for individuals except in the law. Pedagogies of discouragement cannot withstand the contemporary defense of right. As long as abortion continues to occupy a controversial place in American life, its acceptance and discouragement will go hand in hand. This is its cultural legacy and the doctor's dilemma.

Appendix:
Methodology
and Interview
Schedules

Methodology

My entrée to Daleton's obstetricians and gynecologists was helped considerably by several physicians who practiced in other specialties there. I also talked to representatives of the local Planned Parenthood office, who familiarized me with the politics of family planning in the community. My initial interview project took place over five months in mid-1978. After the first round of interviews I spoke again with several doctors who had expressed an interest in knowing what I had learned from their colleagues. I used these second occasions to ask questions that had arisen during the course of my fieldwork.

Over time the community of practitioners changed. By 1981, two of the physicians I had interviewed had died, and several new doctors had joined established groups. I again contacted physicians in Daleton who were willing to read my dissertation. This served as an opportunity to confirm what I had already written, but it also became an occasion for the physicians to express themselves further and at greater length about matters other than abortion. These interviews were less structured, and all but one doctor gave me permission to tape-record what was said. Because there were three hospitals in Daleton, I sought in the final stages of the project to talk with physicians in each of these constellations of medical practice in order to confirm the accuracy of my original reporting.

The most difficult methodological problem I faced was the reluctance of several physicians to talk in any detail about their attitudes and practices. One, as I have mentioned elsewhere, refused to be interviewed despite my repeated attempts. Another was willing to talk by telephone but not in person. What I took as investigating some took as prying. Their reticence was partly due to the sensitive nature of many of the questions I asked. One physician refused to discuss his wife's views about abortion. Another told me directly that I asked too many questions about abortion and that my phone "pitch" inviting myself to his office had not been fully candid. Another informed me that abortion was a "hot topic" in his group, and he explicitly asked me not to repeat his views to any of his colleagues.

In the interview schedules that follow, certain questions listed are not addressed in this book. Questioning physicians about their medical practices led progressively to a refocusing of topics about what each of us thought was important to discuss. I obtained biographical data about all the physicians, but I did not cover the entire range of questions that are presented here with every physician who was interviewed. I did not discourage physicians who were willing to talk extensively about their views of medical practice in Daleton by attempting to seek answers for all the questions I had prepared. Although I initially directed the course of discussions, especially in the follow-up interviews I was led by whatever struck them as most interesting to think out loud about.

The interview schedules thus stand for my initial interests, while my final report shows how those interests were reshaped by the physicians themselves. I admit that I did not "let" this happen; it happened to me. By paying attention to what concerned them most and by pursuing those concerns further at the expense of other ones, I forfeited scientific form for something intrinsically more important to me: I wanted to know what was on their minds and I wanted to hear them talk about themselves and their colleagues. I cannot maintain that the opinions and practices of physicians in Daleton will be found in another community of practitioners. But what I have described here is more than a pattern of practices unique to one time or one place. The dilemma of the professional—to judge and act consistently—was fully revealed in this one community's confrontation with a major moral issue. Inconsistencies in physicians' rationales for handling abortion are hardly to be condemned, for they signal the responses of individual conscience—expedient, anguished, or otherwise—to public demands that the physician take a stand on this issue. How this stand is taken and what its consequences may be for the abortion dilemma and the practice of medicine are subject to revision and reevaluation by those who can report on other experiences with these same matters.

| Interview Schedules

First Interview (April–August 1978)

Name
Date of birth
Marital status
Spouse's birth date
Spouse's occupation
Number of children
    Age/sex
Religion (denomination)
    Spouse, children
Do you regularly attend?
    Alone/with family?
Ethnic background

Father's occupation
    Education
    Religion (denomination)
Mother's occupation
    Education
    Religion (denomination)
Number of brothers and sisters
What is your age in relation to them?

Where were you born?
Where did you primarily grow up?
    (city, town, country)

How did you come to choose medicine as a career?
    When did you make this decision?

Where did you receive your medical education?
    When did you receive your M.D.?
    Where did you do your residency?

How did you come to decide upon this specialty?
    Any previous one(s)?
    Who or what influenced you?

How long have you practiced in this community?
How and why did you decide upon this community?

What community activities do you participate in (for example, school board, bank, and church)?

Are you a current member of the AMA?
  Why or why not?

To what other (medical) professional organizations do you belong?

Which journals do you follow?

Have you ever been formally questioned about your attitudes toward birth
  control, abortion, or family planning?
  If yes, when, where, by whom?

What is your relationship to the Planned Parenthood organization in this
  community?
  How regular is your contact with them?

If you discuss abortion with your spouse, what are her/his views generally?
  (If those views are different from your own, how do you feel about that?)

What types of contraception do you mostly prescribe?
  How do you determine what types are most appropriate for each patient?

Do you think there are contraceptives that are abortive rather than concep-
  tion-preventing?
  Do patients ever ask you about this distinction?

How do *you* define abortion?

Are you aware of any other physicians in the community, besides members
  of your specialty, who perform abortions?

Can you recall the circumstances of the most "medically" troublesome abortion you ever performed?

Have you ever refused an abortion to a woman requesting one?
  What happened? To whom was she referred?

Could you speculate on why abortion is so widely practiced (if you think
  it is), even when birth control is available?
  In other words, what prevents men and women from using contraception?

How do you ideally envision the participation of men and women in the
  use of contraceptives?
  What role should men play?

How do you feel about seeing only one half or side of a sexual relationship,
  when there are more than simply medical problems?

How familiar are you with the Supreme Court rulings that brought about
  the present conformity of abortion laws throughout the United States?
  Can you tell me the basic issues in *Roe v. Wade* and *Doe v. Bolton?*

Why do only ob/gyns perform abortions, when the court explicitly states that any licensed M.D. may do so?

At the present time, there appear to be two social movements in America specifically devoted to the abortion issue. Have you ever experienced any form of pressure from either the proponents of pro-choice or their opponents, the pro-life movement?

What do you believe the physician's place ought to be in the public controversy over abortion?

What are your feelings about the pro-life attempt to amend the U.S. Constitution?

Where do you stand on the matter of federal funding to subsidize abortions for women who are unable to afford them?

Do you think that federal funds should be denied to hospitals that refuse to allow abortions or sterilizations on the basis of moral or religious beliefs?

Although the swearing to uphold the Hippocratic oath is no longer required in order to receive a medical degree (this is true of many medical schools, Harvard for instance, since 1969), how do you reconcile the liberalizing of abortion with Hippocrates' injunction against it? ("I will not give a woman a pessary to cause abortion.") Did you take the oath?

Are you familiar with any physicians or hospital personnel who will not participate in abortion and who are not Catholic?

May I ask who they are and what reasons they give for their views?

In your clinical experience, have you ever seen a woman who has had difficulties with infertility or premature delivery and who had undergone a previous abortion? (In a report published in *Obstetrical and Gynecological Survey* [30:629–31, 1975] the authors reported that infertility and premature births are becoming the "ravages of the liberal abortion era." Had you heard of this?

What do you make of it?

Do you or would you advise women seeking abortions of this claim?

Are there contraceptives which you prescribe that you personally consider less than perfectly safe?

Do you advise patients to whom you prescribe these contraceptives of your thoughts on such matters?

How would you respond to legislation authorizing nonphysicians to perform abortions?

Have you ever used or heard of any physician using paramedic personnel for performing abortions?

Are you familiar with the name of Dr. Bernard N. Nathanson?
What do you make of him?

When polls of physicians' attitudes toward abortion were conducted in the late 1960s and early 1970s, they were asked to react to "varying situations" in which they would or would not approve abortion. For instance, a study done in 1976 for the *American Journal of Public Health* asked for physicians' responses to these varying situations. I would like to probe with you more deeply these various situations. Put yourself in the position of a physician faced with any of these various circumstances, even if you have not been:

(a) The pregnancy or childbirth is a threat to the woman's life.

What kinds of conditions would you consider threatening?
Have you ever had such a case?

(b) There is a risk of congenital abnormality.

How significant a risk would there have to be?
How would you diagnose such a risk?
Under what circumstances do you have women tested for such conditions?
Have you ever had any cases in which you performed an abortion because there was, in your mind, significant risk of congenital abnormality?
Describe the circumstances.

(c) The pregnancy or childbirth is a threat to the woman's physical health.

What threats to physical health have you diagnosed which persuaded you that an abortion was necessary?
What threats might persuade you?

(d) The pregnancy is the result of rape or incest.

Have you ever performed an abortion for either of these reasons?
Is there any case that stands out in your mind as troubling? (Your own or someone else's?)
Could you describe it?

(e) The pregnancy or childbirth is a threat to a woman's mental health.

Have you ever performed an abortion for this reason?
What were the circumstances?
Upon whose diagnosis did you rely for determining what a threat to mental health is?
Did you perform abortions when psychiatric indications were required for any therapeutic abortions performed?
Do psychiatrists play any role in your decision to perform abortions today?

(f) Being unmarried would be a problem.

Would you explore how serious a problem?
Have you ever had such a case?

(g) The woman does not want the child.

Would you ask if she ever wants children?
If she never wanted children, would you advise abortion and sterilization?
Have you ever had such a case?

(h) The woman is financially unable to support the child.

Have you ever had such a case?
If you did, would you or did you propose ways to find finances?
Would you draw a line (say in terms of income) over which this reason would no longer be convincing to you?

(i) The woman is too old to have the child.

In your mind, how old is too old?
Have you ever had such a case?

(j) The woman is too young to have the child.

Would you distinguish between her judgment, your judgment, or her parents' judgment, if they were involved?
Have you ever had a case in which the parents were involved?
In your mind, how young is too young?

(k) The woman's education or career would be disrupted.

Would you explore how disrupted?
Have you ever had such a case?

(l) The pregnancy is the result of contraceptive failure.

Have you ever had such a case?

(m) The pregnancy is the result of contraceptive failure and the contraception was prescribed by the physician being asked to perform the abortion.

Have you ever had such a case?
Is there any particular contraceptive you know that seems to fail more than others?

(n) The pregnancy is the result of failure to use contraception.

Have you ever had such a case?
Do you have any other feelings about this particular problem?

(o) The pregnancy is not the result of rape, but the woman is not certain who the father is.

Have you ever had such a case?

(p) The woman requests the abortion because her husband (or whoever the father is) asks that she have an abortion.
Have you ever had such a case?

(q) The woman requests the abortion and refuses to give any reason.
Have you ever had such a case?

(r) The pregnancy is in the first trimester.

(s) The pregnancy is in the second trimester.

(t) The pregnancy is in the third trimester.
Have you ever had such a case?

Have you ever been faced with or heard about women who have sought repeated abortions?
What was or would be your reaction to this situation?

How would you relate the population problem with the practice of abortion?

In your view and experience, who have abortions? (married, unmarried, young, poor, etc.)

I would like to ask some questions about that which is aborted in abortion. One way of focusing on the problem of when life begins is through the problem of viability.
Do you have a definition for this term?

With potential developments in the technology of prenatal care, how will you, as a physician, face the prospect that any abortion one performs may involve a viable fetus?

Do you distinguish, in the case of the fetus, between life and human life?

Are you familiar with or do you perform menstrual extraction, regulation, or aspiration?
What are your views on this procedure?

At some point, pharmaceutical solutions to unwanted conceptions may become a reality, at least for the first trimester.
Do you think that abortion practice (or your abortion practice) will decrease dramatically in such an event? Why or why not?

Are you familiar with any research being performed upon fetuses in or outside the community?

Have you ever been approached and asked to provide fetuses for such research?

Do you recommend amniocentesis for the purpose of diagnosing genetic disorders in the fetus?
How often?

Who else in the community uses it?

Suppose a child were born deformed; could you ever see a suit being brought against you for not having taken precautions (namely, amniocentesis and abortion) against such a possibility?

Would you perform an abortion if you knew the reason why it was requested was that the woman or couple did not want a child of a certain sex?

What techniques for abortion do you generally use?

How much do you charge for an abortion?

Follow-up Interview (June–September 1981)

Would you say that in the last three years, requests made of you for abortions have increased, decreased, or remained the same?
How do you account for the change, if any?

Have you been following the congressional hearings on the so-called human life bill?
What are your thoughts about it?

A state proposal "to make convenience abortions as inconvenient as possible" (as one lawmaker put it) would affect physicians directly. What are your reactions to some of the following stipulations in that proposal?

(a) required labeling of any substance or device that induces abortion as an abortifacient. The IUD is included.

(b) birth and death certificates for all aborted fetuses at any stage of gestation.

(c) restructuring all health insurance laws to have separate premiums for abortion coverage.

(d) parental consent for minors seeking abortion.

(e) notification to the father.

(f) informed consent—physician required to explain in detail the developmental growth of the fetus, the abortion technique to be used, and its effect on the fetus.

(g) second-trimester and third-trimester abortions: method least damaging to the fetus to be used.

(h) waiting period—no abortion could be performed prior to seventy-two hours after signing an informed consent form.

(i) wrongful life suits—physicians could not be held liable for *not* aborting a fetus born with birth defects, or not using amniocentesis.

(j) abortion clinics: stringent reporting requirements—release of information on facilities, who the physicians are, the number of abortions they perform. Health Department does not release such information at present.

How do you at present regard the issue of abortion as a right?
In other words, should abortion not only be considered a woman's right but also an essential part of health and welfare policy?

Do you think that recent developments, such as the election of Ronald Reagan or the rise of the Moral Majority, have discouraged you from performing abortions?

What do physicians have to contribute to the debate in Congress about the definitions of *human life* and *personhood*?

What was your reaction to new congressional provisions that allow federal funds for abortions only when the mother's life is in danger—in effect, the rape and incest clauses have been dropped?

Have you seen, do you expect to see, or have you heard from others who have seen a rise in maternal mortality and morbidity as a result of federal restrictions on abortion funding?

Do you think that abortion is going to be made illegal again?

How would you characterize the mood in this community regarding family planning and abortion?
Has it improved or gotten worse since 1978?

How are you affected, if you are, by local groups opposed to abortion?

Have there been any changes in hospital policy regarding abortion?

Have you had any part in the recent controversies at United Way?

How can such matters be resolved within the community?
Do physicians have a part to play?

Would you consider any of the work you are doing, or any of the work that you know your colleagues are doing in obstetrics and gynecology, experimental in nature; or would you describe your work as basically clinical? (I am trying to get your impressions here about recent controversies concerning breast surgery, the pill, diethylstilbestrol, and other such topics.)

How do you assure yourself that what you are doing does not have possible long-term effects about which little is known?

What about male birth control in this country?

What do you think of test-tube baby research?
Have you made any referrals to clinics offering this service?

Do you continue to refer patients requesting abortions?

Do you see any difference between abortion referrals and other types of referral, since you could competently perform an abortion?

To whom do you refer?

What are the present charges for abortion?

Notes

Preface

1. Carol Joffe has written that "what abortion counselors most want from their clients is an acknowledgment of the normally problematic nature of abortion, but clients are less and less willing to grant this. The feminist ideology, which served abortion counselors well in the period before legalization, seems unsuited to making such a demand—indeed any demand—on abortion clients" (1978:113).

2. The medical specialty known as obstetrics and gynecology has its origins in the rise of professional medicine in the late nineteenth and early twentieth centuries. Throughout this book I refer to practitioners who assume the multiple responsibilities of this specialty, including "the patient's prenatal period; her pregnancy and its complications, including care of the patient and the fetus; obstetric procedures during parturition; the postpartum period; and considerations of infertility, contraception, and avoidance of disease and injury to mother and child" (Fineberg *et al.*, 1984:8; see also Arney, 1982.)

Chapter 1 Abortion as a Medical Responsibility

1. Both Mohr and Paul Starr (1982) understate the importance of the scientific ethos in nineteenth-century medicine. Yet it undoubtedly inspired efforts to restrict access to medical schools, to establish medical societies around the country, and to require state licensing of physicians. Starr's work, like Mohr's, offers a persuasive analysis of professionalization, attributing it to the restructuring of the social bases of medical practice, but both books de-emphasize the ideology of scientific vocation that inspired this restructuring and that continues, despite the introduction of corporate management techniques into medical practice, to inform the physician's calling to medicine.

2. The visual realities of birth and abortion are examined in more detail in chaps. 4 and 5.

3. Only one of the abortions in Simons' study was classified as therapeutic.

4. The use of historical analogies to underwrite a moral crusade is particularly

evident in the arguments made by those in the right-to-life movement. The legal standing of Jews and others under the Third Reich is often compared with the standing of the unborn after *Roe v. Wade* (see Koop, 1976). Milton C. Sernett has examined in detail another analogy between "fetal personhood" and American blacks under slavery, or "more precisely between the implications of *Roe v. Wade* and *Dred Scott v. Sanford*" (1980:461; see also Thomas, 1984).

5. I take the formulation of the terms *medicalization* and *demedicalization* from Renée C. Fox, 1979:465–483. In the case of abortion, one might view the decision to abort as entirely a medical responsibility (complete medicalization) or as entirely the patient's choice (complete demedicalization). Clearly it is neither.

6. See Alan F. Guttmacher, "The Shrinking Non-Psychiatric Indications for Therapeutic Abortion" (1954). Guttmacher's article was published in Harold Rosen's *Therapeutic Abortion* (1954). Rosen's book opened the public discussion of abortion in the 1950s, and Guttmacher encouraged this by asserting that abortion was no longer exclusively, or even primarily, a medical problem. This had been anticipated in the work of Taussig and others (Callahan, 1970:27–47). In an "Obstetrical Foreword" to Rosen's book, Nicholson J. Eastman assessed the matter in nearly the opposite way from those calling for the liberalization of medical indications and the law: "The feeling is growing apparently among the leaders in psychiatry that therapeutic abortion on psychiatric grounds is often a double edged sword and frequently carries with it a degree of emotional trauma far exceeding that which would have been sustained by continuation of pregnancy" (Eastman, 1954:xxi). It is remarkable how Eastman's conclusion is exactly reversed in contemporary rationales for the resort to abortion (see also Eastman, 1967).

7. See Olson *et al.*, 1943; Dannreuther, 1946; Perlmutter, 1947; Tietze, 1948, 1950; Russell, 1951; J. G. Moore and Randall, 1952; Heffernan and Lynch, 1953; Thornton, Jr., 1953; Colpitts, 1954; Stephenson, 1954; Nelson and Hunter, 1957; Hanley, 1958; Scherman, 1958; Routledge *et al.*, 1961; Boulas *et al.*, 1962; Lederman, 1963; Hammond, 1964; Hall, 1965; Lohner, 1966; Niswander *et al.*, 1966; and Hall, 1967.

Chapter 2 The Physician in the Abortion Controversy

1. The literature on feminism and abortion is extensive. For a review of various perspectives, see Vetterling-Braggin *et al.*, 1977:377–445, and Petchesky, 1984. See also Firestone, 1970; Richards, 1980; and Harrison, 1983. For recent philosophical discussion that criticizes the radical feminist defense of abortion, see McMillan, 1982.

2. The logic of medical indications for abortion, which had evolved on the assumption that abortion was to be used as a last resort when pregnancy posed a direct threat to the mother's life, was not at stake in the Court's reference to medical knowledge. Instead, restrictions on it were said to be based entirely on the danger it posed to the woman.

3. After the Supreme Court rulings in 1973, a prominent spokesman for the medical profession, Dr. John H. Knowles, who was then president of the Rockefeller Foundation, proposed a more aggressive policy to deal with the inevitable inequities in the provision of abortion services. Knowles's concern was to maximize the medical safety of abortions. He also believed that "the moral and socioeconomic cost of abortion services has to be weighed against the moral and socioeconomic cost of unwanted infants. I have no reason to doubt the wisdom of the Supreme Court in its decision" (1974:18). Knowles's weighing of the costs was an elegant resignation to the status quo. This resignation has expressed itself in less intellectually refined ways, but the similarity in the weighing of "costs" between elites and underclass is too powerful to go sociologically un-remarked. See the *New York Times,* July 5, 1979, p. A15. The headline read: "Chicagoan Given 40 to 80 Years in Starvation Death of Daughters." "CHICAGO, July 4 (AP)—A 27-year old South Side man has been sentenced to 40 to 80 years in prison for the starvation deaths of his two young daughters. 'Why did you ever have children in the first place?' Circuit Judge James Bailey asked yesterday at a sentence hearing. 'My wife wasn't into abortion,' replied Dwight Battles, convicted June 1 of the murders."

4. See also Ramsey, 1978:43–93. For two other early reports by physicians on the tremendous demand for abortion following its legalization, see Julienne, 1970, and Weisman, 1972.

5. In the case of abortion, the exercise of privacy requires considerable interdependence, perhaps more than any other means of birth control including contraceptive sterilization. At least four types of individuality can be directly implicated in determining how this privacy is understood: the maternal, the fetal, the paternal, and the professional. The vast ideological struggle that ensues over the issue of abortion as a private and public matter is derived from the different rights assigned to three types of individuality. For a survey of the paternal response to abortion, see Shostak *et al.,* 1984.

6. For an interview with Nathanson that traces his changing views, see Norma Rosen, 1977. For another interview with Nathanson and Harriet Pilpel, see Donahue, 1979. See also Nathanson and Ostling, 1979, and Nathanson, 1983. For a review of Nathanson and Ostling, 1979, see Imber, 1980.

7. Thomson's argument emphasized that abortion must remain an individual decision, but one tempered by some acknowledgment of the separate, but dependent, existence of the fetus and of the specific circumstances under which the abortion is sought. In this sense, despite Thomson's reference to traditions of religious thinking on the subject, her entire effort has ample precedent in, and far greater affinity with, medical thinking. The physician's role, however, is summarily reduced to the expression "third party," whose sole interest in the matter is a technical one because "things being as they are, there isn't much a woman can do to abort herself" (ibid.). In this single observation is contained the dilemma of abortion from the sociomedical perspective; for insofar as it has not yet been made private by an efficient, effective, and safe do-it-yourself technology, it directly implicates others in its performance. The kind of privacy afforded by such technological innovation would finally alter the social reality that gave rise to and continues to provoke public debate. The question of control, which Thomson and other philosophers address with their imaginary analogies, would no longer depend so intimately on the existence of a third party.

8. See Tooley, 1983, in particular his response to Wertheimer's (1977) assessment of his position on pp. 309–310.

9. It remains for a sociology of medical ethics to explain why the act of abortion is examined by philosophers as a matter of rights or as a disputation on the nature of personhood. The explanation, I believe, is contained in the philosopher's inclination to construct problems that can be solved by rational cognition, as if all human problems were a matter of *thinking correctly*. For discussions of the role of the unconscious in matters pertaining to birth control, see Flugel, 1947, and Devereux, 1976. As to thinking correctly, the abortion issue has mobilized sides in such a way that politically correct thinking has become the standard by which public debate is conducted, thus forcing an uncritical opposition or defense of the procedure. Who imagines that there could be *no* reason for abortion or that *all* reasons (including no reason at all) must be equally respected because every circumstance is unique to every individual? Those on one side know no exceptions; those on the other side know nothing but exceptions. If abortion remains a moral problem, even to those who advocate its remission in every circumstance, it is because moral problems are about the *meaning* of choice, not about its uncritical defense or opposition (see Ramsey, 1978, and Kass, 1985).

Chapter 3 Medical Practice and Family Planning in Daleton

1. With the help of the local medical society, I was able to obtain biographical data (e.g., age, year of graduation from medical school, and place of residency) about the one physician who refused to be interviewed.

2. This is generally the case among physicians beginning private practice. See Mechanic, 1979:178.

3. These guidelines are published by and available from the American Board of Obstetrics and Gynecology, Inc., 100 Meadow Road, Buffalo, N.Y. 14216.

4. I am not arguing that Sanger's rhetoric coincided even at that time with medical expectations about who should use birth control. In his essay "Is There a Special Sex Life of the Unmarried Adult?" Dr. Ira S. Wile, who was then lecturer on disorders of conduct and personality at Columbia University, quoted approvingly from T. W. Galloway's *Sex and Social Health (1924): "On purely physiological* grounds there is no reason why temperate sex intercourse should be allowed in marriage and denied to the unmarried. Marriage makes no difference whatever in physiology. *It is to be frankly admitted therefore that any grounds for sexual abstinence of people, younger or older, are not biological but social, esthetic and ethical.* This does not mean that they are any less compelling." Wile went on to point out, "They are less compelling than a decade ago" (1934:45).

5. For reports on illegally performed abortions, see Dr. X as Told to Lucy Freeman, 1962; Dares, 1963; Lee, 1969; and Polgar and Fried, 1976.

6. For an assessment of menstrual regulation, see Edelman and Berger, 1981. Dilation and curettage and other methods for early abortion are described in more detail in chap. 4.

Chapter 4 The First-Trimester Abortion

1. Although one of these six Catholic physicians refused to be interviewed, I confirmed through other physicians that he did not perform elective abortions, at least not in Daleton.

2. D & C is used not only for termination of pregnancy. Fineberg *et al.* have noted that "the American College of Obstetricians and Gynecologists has not identified specific standards of care governing the performance of a D & C." Its use "as a diagnostic tool and as a treatment for certain gynecological and obstetrical conditions" is widespread (1984:516–517).

3. The expression "dirty work" was used by Dr. Adams. For a sociological assessment of the idea, see Hughes, 1971:343–345.

4. On June 15, 1983, the Supreme Court, in *Akron v. Akron Center for Reproductive Health* (No. 81-746), ruled that second-trimester abortions no longer had to be performed exclusively in hospitals, as had been required by law since 1973. The technical innovation of D & E (dilation and evacuation), discussed further in chap. 5, can now be used in non-ambulatory clinics, making the second-trimester abortion from a legal point of view as routine as the first-trimester one.

5. Sarvis and Rodman noted very early on in the political debate over abortion that "the partisan use of evidence forms one of the most colorful

chapters in the abortion controversy" (1974:106). That chapter is hardly at an end. In the 1950s and 1960s, researchers sought to determine whether significant psychological harm was associated with induced abortion. Zimmerman (1977) has criticized the narrow psychological focus of this research. The research of the 1970s and 1980s has been, in many respects, even more reductionistic, insofar as it concentrates on the physiological harm associated with induced abortion. The discussion of what types of harm occur has evolved toward a presumably more "scientific" form. The irony of this evolution rests on the assumption that in order to talk more scientifically about harm from abortions, one can no longer talk about the persons who perform and undergo them. Indeed, all research on abortion, including the epidemiological, is immediately suspect (to one side or the other) because "evidence" has an implicit rhetorical function: to persuade us to approve or disapprove of abortion practice. See also Brennan, 1974.

6. Bolognese and Corson have discussed a variety of medical indications for abortion (e.g., chronic heart disease, severe hypertension, and renal diseases) and conclude: "Because of the wide range of medical advances affecting obstetrics and the improved health status of women in the reproductive age, therapeutic abortions now performed for medical indications are uncommon. . . . Obviously, each case must be evaluated individually with consultation from a specialist in the discipline involved. The final decision rests with the couple and their desire for children with full knowledge of the risks to the mother" (1975:168).

7. This quotation is taken directly from a state Medical Assistance Memorandum entitled "Reimbursement for Abortions." The full citation of the Supreme Court ruling is *Beal v. Doe,* 432 U.S. 438 (1977).

8. Nathanson and Becker have offered a sociological explanation (exemplified here in the views and actions of Dr. Adams) for the liberal physician's participation in abortion: "These are physicians with largely middle-class and predominately white practices. Their comments in connection with fee policies reflect a generally suspicious and defensive attitude toward any patient who is personally unknown or is referred by an unknown physician. The patient management procedures of these physicians, we would suggest, are the outcome of an abortion practice limited to women of their own social status with whom a prior personal or professional relationship exists. This relationship precludes the need for consent or for payment in advance; the abortion is done mainly as an accommodation. Medicaid patients are not accepted because they do not meet the physician's interpersonal criteria for abortion performance" (1977:163). What needs to be considered further, following Nathanson

and Becker's analysis, is whether the social class of physicians explains fully why some doctors respond to patient requests for abortion in this way. Is there anything significant about abortion itself and about the practice of medicine in a community that might explain their responses? If not, then one is left with a more obvious generalization: that the social class of physicians (i.e., private practice itself) determines to a large extent the kinds of patients they will be willing to see for any treatment or procedure, including abortion (see also LoSciuto *et al.,* 1972; Nathanson and Becker, 1978; and P. L. Stewart, 1978).

9. Several Daleton physicians restricted their medical practices to gynecology only. Some were older, solo practitioners who preferred to avoid the prospect of getting up in the middle of the night to perform a delivery. Others were in group practices that were able to support a specialist in gynecology.

10. Nathanson and Becker (1980) reached a similar conclusion about the pivotal role of the physician in determining access to abortion (see also Nathanson and Becker, 1981.) Many physicians will probably remain impervious to demands that are not viewed as reasonable improvements in the scientific treatment of disease. The consequence of the simultaneous medicalization and demedicalization of abortion is that reasonable improvements in its technical performance have been adopted while the demand that it be more equitably provided has not (see Borders and Cutright, 1979).

11. The Daleton yellow pages listed obstetrics and gynecology in the Physicians & Surgeons Medical, M.D. Specialty Guide. All Daleton's obstetrician/gynecologists listed their names. Beneath their names, many added "Office Hours by Appointment Only."

12. Dr. Vincent is discussed further in chap. 6.

13. See n. 4 above. Dilation and evacuation and other methods for midtrimester abortion are described further in chap. 5.

14. Lindheim and Cotterill (1978) have argued that residency programs and the obstetrician/gynecologists who run them can be made more responsive to the provision of abortion services. This may be true in some programs, but socialization in residency may not persist as strongly as some may hope after a physician moves into private practice.

Chapter 5 The Second-Trimester Abortion

1. For two studies comparing prostaglandins with hypertonic saline solution, see Bygdeman, 1978, and Cates, Jr., *et al.,* 1978. For a discussion of prostaglandins, see Bygdeman, 1981.

2. The rapid acceptance of D & E is attributable to studies comparing it

with prostaglandins. To follow the evolution of this innovation, see Grimes *et al.*, 1977a, 1977b; Benditt, 1979; Grimes *et al.*, 1980; Cadesky *et al.*, 1981; and Stubblefield, 1981. For an overview of the concept of innovation, see Rogers, 1983.

3. Lewit quoted from Nancy B. Kaltreider, "Psychological Impact on Patients and Staff," in Berger *et al.*, 1981:239–249. David Grimes *et al.* expressed a similar expectation when they wrote: "Greater technical and emotional involvement in midtrimester abortion appears to be a worthwhile price for physicians to pay, however, when the gains to women in safety, speed, comfort, and acceptance are so large" (1980:789–790). According to Carl W. Tyler, Jr., "By showing that D & E is a safe method of second-trimester abortion, epidemiology has made worthwhile contributions to the practice of obstetrics and gynecology over the past decade. The potential for epidemiology to favorably influence other areas of reproductive medicine is substantial but, at present, unrealized" (1981:468). See also Rooks and Cates, Jr., 1977.

4. Carl Scheffel defined *medical jurisprudence* (under which obstetric jurisprudence would be subsumed) as "that branch of science which shows how the law affects the practice of medicine." Legal or forensic medicine "applies to the manner in which medical science affects legal practice and aids in furthering justice" (1931:ix).

5. Harry Harris has written: "There is something paradoxical about a situation in which a fetus may be judged at one point in time as a suitable candidate for abortion, and a very few weeks later, if prematurely born, as a candidate for the application of the powerful modern machinery of intensive care" (1975:78).

6. See *State Definitions and Reporting Requirements for Live Births, Fetal Deaths, and Induced Terminations of Pregnancy* (1981). This report gives a state-by-state account of (1) current definitions of live birth, fetal death (stillbirth), and induced termination of pregnancy; (2) the period of gestation at which a fetal death must be reported; and (3) when induced termination of pregnancy must be reported. In order to preserve the anonymity of Daleton, I do not refer to specific state regulations contained in this report. It is nevertheless useful for demonstrating the inconsistencies in state laws that have made second-trimester abortions more problematic than first-trimester ones for physicians.

7. I am referring, e.g., to the indictment of Dr. Kenneth Edelin for reckless manslaughter in late 1973. Dr. Edelin had performed a hysterotomy. For a thorough and important account of Edelin's trial and of the subsequent reversal of his conviction, see Ramsey, 1978:94–142. See also Wagner, 1978, and Stroh and Hinman, 1976.

8. Hall was editor of an influential two-volume work entitled *Abortion in a Changing World* (1970). At the time, he was associate professor of clinical obstetrics and gynecology at Columbia University College of Physicians and Surgeons, and president of the Association for the Study of Abortion, which was dissolved, according to the *Times,* after the 1973 Supreme Court rulings. See his reflections on these rulings (1973).

Chapter 6 Innovation and the Refuge of Private Practice

1. Conversations reviewed here with Dr. Vincent were conducted during a follow-up interview two years after the first one.
2. Eliot Freidson has given a pertinent description of the sources of conflict among physicians in group practice: "The ground of biography was pervasive in explanations of why, after perceiving offense, the perceiver did not attempt to change the behavior of the offender. Changing ingrained habits being impossible, once a person is out in practice and is set in his ways, rather little can be done to either persuade him of his error or otherwise redirect his habits" (1980:231).
3. David Daube has discussed the phenomenon of the ascetic physician: "As a layman, it is proper for me to stress the cost of some therapies to the doctor. A few weeks ago I passed through an American city. I had lunch with friends from Classics and Law, and we were joined by the professor of surgery. Excellent, un-American wine was produced. I noticed that the surgeon declined it and as I knew him to be healthy and fond of good food and drink I questioned him. It turned out that there was a baby in his hospital with kidney trouble. He could be kept alive for some six months, within which it was hoped to find a kidney that might be given him. If a suitable kidney offered, the transplantation would have to be performed without delay. So the professor kept in continuous touch with the hospital and radically abstained from alcohol. That man, a twentieth-century version of St. Francis, did not pause to enquire into food-production per head of population or the gain or loss to the body politic. The baby needed him" (1967:1239).
4. Some physicians listed their home numbers under their own names, and others under their wives' initials.
5. The discussion of uncertainty in this section is indebted to Fox, 1980.
6. John C. Fletcher has written: "Prenatal diagnosis of disease or malformation in the fetus *in utero* was applied to as many as 40,000 pregnancies in the United States by 1978. In 1978 alone, 15,000 of these procedures were done, indicating a recent rapid increase. In the earliest use of amniocentesis, prior to the knowledge of its safety and efficacy, some investigators argued that parents who were not willing to accept abortion

should not be allowed to obtain amniocentesis, because bearing the un-known risks could be justified only by abortion when a diagnosis was positive. Because studies of the safety and technical accuracy of amni-ocentesis have firmly established that the possibilities of fetal death and technical error are each less than 1 percent, this early restriction has been relaxed" (notes not included) (1983:220).

7. For a study of the development of the pill, see Merkin, 1976. See also Seaman and Seaman, 1977.

8. Gordon Horobin has written: "[The physician's] charisma is maintained through the paradox that increasing knowledge and control through sci-ence creates new uncertainties (the more we know, the more we realise how much there is to know). Such an argument runs rather against the more usual one that science, in the long run, reduces uncertainty" (1983:104).

Chapter 7 Beyond the Politics of Abortion

1. For an early medical reaction to abortion clinics in California, see Ford, 1972 (along with "Letter to the Editor," 1973); and see Denes, 1976a and 1976b.

2. It is beyond the scope of this book to assess what kinds of policies for the reduction of abortion might be most successful. There are no doubt many who believe that "better" sex education would reduce the resort to abortion. Unfortunately, those who approve in principle of such ed-ucation are typically drawn to the pro-choice side of the abortion debate while those who disapprove are drawn to the pro-life side. The political division over abortion obfuscates a more fundamental problem about what "control" over reproduction means. If the present provision of re-productive services in this country reflects the ambiguous status of abor-tion as a form of birth control, efforts toward its reduction should be first directed toward a better understanding of the role of primary groups and other mediating institutions, including schools and churches, in mat-ters pertaining to sexuality, birth, and abortion. For an important survey of this kind of effort, see Ooms, 1981.

References

American Law Institute. 1959. Model Penal Code. Tentative draft no. 9, submitted by the council to the members for discussion at the thirty-sixth annual meeting, May 20–23, pp. 146–166. Philadelphia: American Law Institute.

Apfel, Roberta J., and Fisher, Susan M. 1984. *To Do No Harm: DES and the Dilemmas of Modern Medicine.* New Haven: Yale University Press.

Arditti, Rita; Klein, Renate Duelli; and Minden, Shelley. 1984. *Test-Tube Women: What Future for Motherhood?* London: Pandora Press.

Arney, William Ray. 1982. *Power and the Profession of Obstetrics.* Chicago: University of Chicago Press.

Bates, Jerome E., and Zawadzki, Edward S. 1964. *Criminal Abortion: A Study in Medical Sociology.* Springfield, Il.: Charles C Thomas.

Bearle, Beatrice Bishop. 1942. An Analysis of Abortion Deaths in the District of Columbia for the Years 1938, 1939, 1940. *American Journal of Obstetrics and Gynecology* (hereafter cited as AJOG) 43:820–826.

Becker, Howard S., and Geer, Blanche. 1958. The Fate of Idealism in Medical School. *American Sociological Review* 23:50–56.

Behrman, Richard E., and Rosen, Tove S. 1975. Report on Viability and Non-viability of the Fetus. In *Appendix: Research on the Fetus,* for the National Commission for the Protection of Human Subjects of Biomedical and Behavioral Research, pp. 12-1–12-116. Washington, D.C.: U.S. Department of Health, Education and Welfare, DHEW Publication no. (OS) 76-128.

Benditt, John. 1979. Second-Trimester Abortion in the United States. *Family Planning Perspectives* 11:358–361.

Berger, Gary S.; Brenner, William E.; and Keith, Louis G., eds. 1981. *Second-Trimester Abortion: Perspectives after a Decade of Experience.* Boston: John Wright–PSG.

Blake, Judith. 1971. Abortion and Public Opinion: The 1960–1970 Decade. *Science* 171:540–549.

————, and Pinal, Jorge del. 1981. Negativism, Equivocation, and Wobbly Assent: Public "Support" for the Pro-Choice Platform on Abortion. *Demography* 18:309–320.

Bland, P. Brooke, and Montgomery, Thaddeus L. [1932]. 1940. *Practical Obstetrics*. 3d rev. ed. Philadelphia: F. A. Davis.

Bolognese, Ronald J., and Corson, Stephen L. 1975. *Interruption of Pregnancy—A Total Patient Approach*. Baltimore: Williams & Wilkins.

Bondeson, William B.; Engelhardt, Jr., H. Tristram; Spicker, Stuart F.; and Winship, Daniel H., eds. 1983. *Abortion and the Status of the Fetus*. Dordrecht, Holland: D. Reidel.

Borders, Jeff A., and Cutright, Phillips. 1979. Community Determinants of U.S. Legal Abortion Rates. *Family Planning Perspectives* 11:227–233.

Bosk, Charles L. 1979. *Forgive and Remember: Managing Medical Failure*. Chicago: University of Chicago Press.

Boulas, Stanley H.; Preucel, Robert W.; and Moore, John H. 1962. Therapeutic Abortion. *Obstetrics and Gynecology* 19:222–227.

Brennan, William C. 1974. Abortion and the Techniques of Neutralization. *Journal of Health and Social Behavior* 15:358–365.

Brunner, Endre K., and Newton, Louis. 1939. Abortions in Relation to Viable Births in 10,609 Pregnancies. AJOG 38:82–90.

Bygdeman, Marc. 1978. Comparison of Prostaglandin and Hypertonic Saline for Termination of Pregnancy. *Obstetrics and Gynecology* 52:424–429.

————. 1981. Prostaglandins. In Jane E. Hodgson, ed., *Abortion and Sterilization: Medical and Social Aspects*, pp. 333–358. New York: Grune & Stratton.

Cadesky, K. I.; Ravinsky, E.; and Lyons, E. R. 1981. Dilation and Evacuation: A Preferred Method of Midtrimester Abortion. AJOG 139:329–332.

Callahan, Daniel. 1970. *Abortion: Law, Choice and Morality*. New York: Macmillan.

————. 1983. At the Center. *Hastings Center Report* 13:4.

Caplow, Theodore; Bahr, Howard M.; Chadwick, Bruce A.; Hill, Reuben; and Williamson, Margaret Holmes. 1982. *Middletown Families: Fifty Years of Change and Continuity*. Minneapolis: University of Minnesota Press.

Capron, Alexander M.; Lappé, Marc; Murray, Robert F.; Powledge, Tabitha M.; Twiss, Sumner B.; and Bergsma, Daniel. 1979. *Genetic Counseling: Facts, Values, and Norms*. New York: Alan R. Liss.

Cates, Jr., Willard; Grimes, David A.; Schulz, Kenneth F.; Ory, Howard W.; and Tyler, Jr., Carl W. 1978. World Health Organization Studies of Prostaglandins Versus Saline Abortifacients: A Reappraisal. *Obstetrics and Gynecology* 52:493–498.

Centers for Disease Control. 1980. *Abortion Surveillance* [1978]. Washington, D.C.: U.S. Department of Health and Human Services, Public Health Service.

————. 1983. *Abortion Surveillance* [1979–1980]. Washington, D.C.: U.S. Department of Health and Human Services, Public Health Service.

Coleman, Samuel. 1983. *Family Planning in Japanese Society: Traditional Birth Control in a Modern Urban Culture.* Princeton: Princeton University Press.

Colpitts, R. Vernon. 1954. Trends in Therapeutic Abortion. AJOG 68:988–997.

Connery, John. 1977. *Abortion: The Development of the Roman Catholic Perspective.* Chicago: Loyola University Press.

Corson, S. L., Bolognese, R. S., and Merola, J. 1973. Intra-amniotic prostaglandin $F_{2\alpha}$ to induce midtrimester abortion. AJOG 117:27–34.

Cosgrove, Samuel A. 1944. "Reply by Dr. Cosgrove," in Correspondence. AJOG 48:893–895.

————, and Carter, Patricia A. 1944. A Consideration of Therapeutic Abortion. AJOG 48:299–314.

Crossen, H. S. 1943. In Memoriam: Frederick Joseph Taussig, 1872–1943. AJOG 46:623–624.

Dannreuther, Walter T. 1946. Therapeutic Abortion in a General Hospital. AJOG 52:54–65.

Dares, Richard. *I Performed Abortions.* 1963. New York: Carlton Press.

Daube, David. 1967. Sanctity of Life. *Proceedings of the Royal Society of Medicine* 60:1235–1240.

David, Henry P.; Friedman, Herbert L.; van der Tak, Jean; and Sevilla, Marylis, J., eds. 1978. *Abortion in Psychosocial Perspective: Trends in Transnational Research.* New York: Springer.

Denes, Magda. 1976a. Performing Abortions. *Commentary* 62:33–37.

————. 1976b. *In Necessity and Sorrow: Life and Death in an Abortion Hospital.* New York: Basic Books.

Devereux, George. [1955]. 1976. *A Study of Abortion in Primitive Societies.* Rev. ed. New York: International Universities Press.

Donahue, Phil. 1979. Donahue Transcript #11199, November 19, 1979, with Phil Donahue, Bernard Nathanson, and Harriet Pilpel. Cincinnati, Ohio: Multimedia Program Productions.

Eastman, Nicholson J. 1944. "Therapeutic Abortion," in Correspondence. AJOG 48:892–893.

————. 1953. "Editor's Note," following a reprinting of Keith P. Russell, Therapeutic Abortions in California in 1950. *Obstetrical and Gynecological Survey* 8:219.

————. 1954. Obstetrical Foreword. In Harold Rosen, ed., *Therapeutic Abortion,* pp. xix–xxi. New York: Julian Press.

————. 1967. Induced Abortion and Contraception: A Consideration of the Ethical Philosophy in Obstetrics. *Obstetrical and Gynecological Survey* 22:3–11.

Edelman, David A., and Berger, Gary S. 1981. Menstrual Regulation. In Jane E. Hodgson, ed., *Abortion and Sterilization: Medical and Social Aspects.* New York: Grune & Stratton.

Ellis, Havelock. [1910]. 1913. *Studies in the Psychology of Sex.* Vol. 6, *Sex in Relation to Society.* Philadelphia: F. A. Davis.

Field, Mark G. 1956. The Re-legalization of Abortion in Soviet Russia. *New England Journal of Medicine.* 255:421–427.

Fineberg, Keith S.; Peters, J. Douglas; Willson, J. Robert; and Kroll, Donald A. 1984. *Obstetrics/Gynecology and the Law.* Ann Arbor: Health Administration Press.

Firestone, Shulamith. 1970. *The Dialectic of Sex: The Case for Feminist Revolution.* New York: Morrow Quill Paperbacks.

Fletcher, John C. 1983. Ethics and Public Policy: Should Sex Choice Be Discouraged? In Neil G. Bennett, ed., *Sex Selection of Children,* pp. 213–252. New York: Academic Press.

Flugel, J. C. 1947. The Psychology of Birth Control. In *Men and Their Motives,* pp. 1–43. New York: International Universities Press.

Ford, James H. 1972. Mass-Produced, Assembly-Line Abortion: A Prime Example of Unethical, Unscientific Medicine. *California Medicine* 117, no. 5:80–84.

Forrest, Jacqueline Darroch; Sullivan, Ellen; and Tietze, Christopher. 1978. Abortion in the United States, 1976–1977. *Family Planning Perspectives* 10:271–283.

————. 1979a. Abortion 1976–1977: Need and Services in the United States, Each State and Metropolitan Area. New York: Alan Guttmacher Institute.

————. 1979b. Abortion in the United States, 1977–1978. *Family Planning Perspectives* 11:329–341.

Fox, Renée C. 1979. The Medicalization and Demedicalization of American Society. In *Essays in Medical Sociology: Journeys into the Field,* pp. 465–483. New York: John Wiley.

Fox, Renée C., and Swazey, Judith P., 1984. Medical Morality Is Not Bioethics—Medical Ethics in China and the United States. *Perspectives in Biology and Medicine* 27:336–360.

————. 1980. The Evolution of Medical Uncertainty. Millbank Memorial Fund Quarterly/*Health and Society.* 58:1–49.

Freeman, M. G., and Graves, W. L. 1970. Physician Attitudes toward Hospital Abortion in Georgia—1970. *Journal of the Medical Association of Georgia* 59:437–446.

Freidson, Eliot. 1970. *Professional Dominance: The Social Structure of Medical Care.* Chicago: Aldine.

————. [1975]. 1980. *Doctoring Together: A Study of Professional Social Control.* Chicago: University of Chicago Press.

Galloway, T. W. *Sex and Social Health.* 1924. New York: American Social Hygiene Association.

Goldstein, Michael S. 1984a. Abortion as a Medical Career Choice: Entrepreneurs, Community Physicians and Others. *Journal of Health and Social Behavior* 25:211–229.

————. 1984b. "Creating and Controlling a Medical Market: Abortion in Los Angeles after Liberalization." *Social Problems* 31:514–529.

Gordon, Linda. 1976. *Woman's Body, Woman's Right: A Social History of Birth Control in America.* New York: Grossman's.

Grimes, David A.; Schulz, Kenneth F.; Cates, Jr., Willard; and Tyler, Jr., Carl W. 1977a. Mid-Trimester Abortion by Dilatation and Evacuation: A Safe and Practical Alternative. *New England Journal of Medicine* 296:1141–1145.

————. Methods of Midtrimester Abortion: Which Is Safest? *International Journal of Gynaecology and Obstetrics* 15:184–188.

————; Hulka, Jaroslav F.; and McCutchen, Mary E. 1980. Midtrimester Abortion by Dilatation and Evacuation versus Intra-amniotic Instillation of Prostaglandin $F_{2\alpha}$: A Randomized Clinical Trial. AJOG 137:785–790.

Grisez, Germain. 1970. *Abortion: The Myths, the Realities, and the Arguments.* New York: Corpus Books.

Guttmacher, Alan F. 1954. The Shrinking Non-Psychiatric Indications for Therapeutic Abortion. In Harold Rosen, ed., *Therapeutic Abortion,* pp. 12–21. New York: Julian Press.

Hall, Robert E. 1965. Therapeutic Abortion, Sterilization and Contraception. AJOG 91:518–532.

————. 1967. Abortion in American Hospitals. *American Journal of Public Health* 57:1933–36.

————, ed. 1970. *Abortion in a Changing World.* 2 vols. New York: Columbia University Press.

————. 1971. Abortion: Physician and Hospital Attitudes. *American Journal of Public Health* 61:517–519.

————. 1973. The Supreme Court Decision on Abortion. AJOG 116:1–8.

————. 1984. Letter to the Editor. "Deadline for Abortion." *New York Times,* February 19, p. E18.

Hamilton, Virginia Clay. 1940. Some Sociologic and Psychologic Observations on Abortion. AJOG 39:919–928.

————. 1941a. II. The Clinical and Laboratory Differentiation of Spontaneous and Induced Abortion. AJOG 41:61–69.

———. 1941b. III. Medical Status and Psychologic Attitude of Patients Following Abortion. AJOG 41:285–288.

Hammond, Howard. 1964. Therapeutic Abortion: Ten Years' Experience with Hospital Committee Control. AJOG 89:349–355.

Hanley, Bernard J. 1958. The Rights of the Unborn Child. *Obstetrical and Gynecological Survey* 13:839–841.

Harris, Harry. 1975. *Prenatal Diagnosis and Selective Abortion.* Cambridge: Harvard University Press.

The Harris Survey Yearbook of Public Opinion: 1972, A Compendium of Current American Attitudes. 1976a. New York: Louis Harris and Associates.

The Harris Survey Yearbook of Public Opinion: 1973, A Compendium of Current American Attitudes. 1976b. New York: Louis Harris and Associates.

Harrison, Beverly Wildung. 1983. *Our Right to Choose: Toward a New Ethic of Abortion.* Boston: Beacon Press.

Heffernan, Roy J., and Lynch, William A. 1953. What Is the Status of Therapeutic Abortion in Modern Obstetrics? AJOG 66:335–345.

Hern, Warren M. 1984. *Abortion Practice.* Philadelphia: J. B. Lippincott.

Hesseltine, H. Close; Adair, F. L.; and Boynton, M. W. 1940. Limitation of Human Reproduction: Therapeutic Abortion. AJOG 39:549–561.

Hilgers, Thomas W., and Horan, Dennis J., eds. 1972. *Abortion and Social Justice.* New York: Sheed & Ward.

———; Horan, Dennis J.; and Mall, David, eds. 1981. *New Perspectives on Human Abortion.* Frederick, Md.: University Publications of America.

Hill, Era L., and Eliot, Johan W. 1972. Black Physicians' Experience with Abortion Requests and Opinion about Abortion Law Change in Michigan. *Journal of the National Medical Association* 64:52–58.

Hogue, Carol J. Rowland; Cates, Jr., Willard; and Tietze, Christopher. 1983. Impact of Vacuum Aspiration Abortion on Future Childbearing: A Review. *Family Planning Perspectives* 15:119–126.

Horobin, Gordon. 1983. Professional Mystery: The Maintenance of Charisma in General Practice. In Robert Dingwall and Philip Lewis, eds., *The Sociology of the Professions: Lawyers, Doctors and Others,* pp. 84–105. London: Macmillan.

Hughes, Everett. 1971. *The Sociological Eye: Selected Papers on Work, Self, and Society.* Chicago: Aldine.

Illich, Ivan. 1976. *Medical Nemesis: The Expropriation of Health.* New York: Pantheon.

Imber, Jonathan B. 1979. Sociology and Abortion: Legacies and Strategies. *Contemporary Sociology* 8:825–832.

———. 1980. Abortion and the Equality of Reasons. *Hastings Center Report* 10, no. 3:44–45.

————. 1985. The Rhetoric of Responsibility: American Medical Responses to the Legalization of Abortion in the Soviet Union, 1920–1936. Paper delivered to the American Association for the History of Medicine, May 15–18, 1985, Durham, North Carolina.

Jaffe, Frederick S.; Lindheim, Barbara L.; and Lee, Philip R. 1981. *Abortion Politics: Private Morality and Public Policy.* New York: McGraw-Hill.

Jakobovits, Immanuel. 1975. *Jewish Medical Ethics.* New York: Bloch Publishing.

Joffe, Carole. 1978. What Abortion Counselors Want from Their Clients. *Social Problems* 26:112–121.

Journal of the American Medical Association. 1967. 201, no. 7:134.

————. 1984. Drug Use in the US in 1981. 251:1293–1297.

Julienne, Mark. 1970. Suddenly I'm a Legal Abortionist. *Medical Economics* 47, no. 25:93–95; 152–168.

Kass, Leon. 1985. *Toward a More Natural Science: Biology and Human Affairs.* New York: Free Press.

Kennedy, David M. 1970. *Birth Control in America: The Career of Margaret Sanger.* New Haven: Yale University Press.

Knowles, John H. 1974. Public Policy on Abortion. *Society* 11, no. 5:15–18.

Koop, Everett C. 1976. *The Right to Live; The Right to Die.* Wheaton, Il.: Tyndale House.

Kopelman, J. Joshua, and Douglas, Gordon W. 1971. Abortions by Resident Physicians in a Municipal Hospital Center. AJOG 111:666–671.

Lederman, J. J. 1963. The Doctor, Abortion, and the Law: A Medicolegal Dilemma. *Obstetrical and Gynecological Survey* 18:59–62.

Lee, Nancy Howell. 1969. *The Search for an Abortionist.* Chicago: University of Chicago Press.

Letter to the Editor. 1973. *California Medicine* 118, no. 3:50–54.

Lewit, Sarah. 1982. D & E Midtrimester Abortion: A Medical Innovation. *Women & Health* 7:49–55.

Lindheim, Barbara L., and Cotterill, Maureen A. 1978. Training in Induced Abortion by Obstetrics and Gynecology Residency Programs. *Family Planning Perspectives* 10:24–28.

Lohner, Richard W. 1966. Therapeutic Abortion in Salt Lake City, 1954–1964. *Obstetrics and Gynecology* 27:665–672.

LoSciuto, Leonard A.; Balin, Howard; and Zahn, Margaret A. 1972. Physicians' Attitudes toward Abortion. *Journal of Reproductive Medicine* 9:70–74.

Luker, Kristin. 1975. *Taking Chances: Abortion and the Decision Not to Contracept.* Berkeley: University of California Press.

————. 1984a. Abortion and the Meaning of Life. In Sidney Callahan and Daniel Callahan, eds., *In Abortion: Understanding Differences*, pp. 25–45. New York: Plenum Press.

————. 1984b. *Abortion and the Politics of Motherhood*. Berkeley: University of California Press.

McDermott, Walsh. 1981. Absence of Indicators of the Influence of Its Physicians on a Society's Health: Impact of Physician Care on Society. *American Journal of Medicine* 70:833–843.

McKeown, Thomas. 1979. *The Role of Medicine: Dream, Mirage or Nemesis?* Princeton: Princeton University Press.

McMillan, Carol. 1982. *Women, Reason and Nature*. Princeton: Princeton University Press.

Maine, Deborah. 1979. Does Abortion Affect Later Pregnancies? *Family Planning Perspectives* 11:98–101.

Marquis, Albert Nelson, ed. 1943. *Who's Who: 1942–43* (vol. 22). Chicago: A. N. Marquis.

————, ed. 1945. *Who's Who: 1944–45* (vol. 23). Chicago: A. N. Marquis.

Mascovich, Paul; Behrstock, Barry; Minor, David; and Colman, Arthur. 1973. Attitudes of Obstetric and Gynecologic Residents toward Abortion. *California Medicine* 119:29–34.

Mechanic, David. 1979. Physicians. In Howard E. Freeman, Sol Levine, and Leo G. Reeder, eds., *Handbook of Medical Sociology*, pp. 177–192. 3d ed. Englewood Cliffs, N.J.: Prentice-Hall.

Merkin, Donald H. 1976. *Pregnancy as a Disease: The Pill in Society*. Port Washington, N.Y.: Kennikat Press.

Modern Medicine. November 3, 1969, Modern Medicine Poll on Socio-medical Issues: Abortion—Homosexual practices—Marihuana. 37, no. 22:18–30.

Mohr, James C. 1978. *Abortion in America: The Origins and Evolution of National Policy*. New York: Oxford University Press.

Moore, J. G., and Randall, J. H. 1952. Trends in Therapeutic Abortion: A Review of 137 Cases. AJOG 63:28–40.

Moore, Thomas V. 1935. *Principles of Ethics*. Philadelphia: J. P. Lippincott.

————. 1940. Moral Aspects of Therapeutic Abortion. AJOG 40:422–428.

Moore-Cavar, Emily Campbell. 1974. *International Inventory of Information on Induced Abortion*. New York: Division of Social and Administrative Sciences, International Institute for the Study of Human Reproduction, Columbia University.

Nadler, Henry L. 1971. Fetal "Indications" for Termination of Pregnancy. In R. Bruce Sloane, ed., *Abortion: Changing Views and Practice*, pp. 92–98. New York: Grune & Stratton.

Nathanson, Bernard N. 1974. Deeper into Abortion. *New England Journal of Medicine.* 291:1189–1190.

———, with Richard N. Ostling. 1979. *Aborting America.* New York: Doubleday.

———. 1983. *The Abortion Papers: Inside the Abortion Mentality.* New York: Frederick Fell.

Nathanson, Constance A., and Becker, Marshall H. 1977. The Influence of Physicians' Attitudes on Abortion Performance, Patient Management and Professional Fees. *Family Planning Perspectives* 9:158–163.

———. 1978. Physician Behavior as a Determinant of Utilization Patterns: The Case of Abortion. *American Journal of Public Health* 68:1104–1114.

———. 1980. Obstetricians' Attitudes and Hospital Abortion Services. *Family Planning Perspectives* 12:26–32.

———. 1981. Professional Norms, Personal Attitudes, and Medical Practice: The Case of Abortion. *Journal of Health and Social Behavior* 22:198–211.

National Abortion Rights Action League (NARAL). 1978. *Newsletter* 10, no. 5.

Nelson, Gunard A., and Hunter, Jr., James S. 1957. Therapeutic Abortion: A Ten-Year Experience. *Obstetrics and Gynecology* 9:284–292.

Nilsson, Lennart. 1977. *A Child Is Born.* Completely rev. ed. New York: Delacorte/Seymour Lawrence.

Niswander, Kenneth R.; Klein, Morton; and Randall, Clyde L. 1966. Therapeutic Abortion: Indications and Techniques. *Obstetrics and Gynecology* 28:124–129.

Noonan, Jr., John T., ed. 1970. *The Morality of Abortion: Legal and Historical Perspectives.* Cambridge: Harvard University Press.

———. 1979. *A Private Choice: Abortion in America in the Seventies.* New York: Free Press.

Olson, Henry J.; Lahmann, A. H.; Mietus, A. C.; and Mitchell, R. M. 1943. The Problem of Abortion. *AJOG* 43:672–678.

Ooms, Theodora. 1981. *Teenage Pregnancy in a Family Context: Implications for Policy.* Philadelphia: Temple University Press.

Perlmutter, Irving K. 1947. Analysis of Therapeutic Abortions, Bellevue Hospital, 1935–1945. *AJOG* 53:1008–1018.

Petchesky, Rosalind Pollack. 1984. *Abortion and Woman's Choice: The State, Sexuality and Reproductive Freedom.* New York: Longman.

Polgar, Steven, and Fried, Ellen S. 1976. The Bad Old Days: Clandestine Abortions among the Poor in New York City before Liberalization of the Abortion Law. *Family Planning Perspectives* 8:125–127.

Potts, Malcolm; Diggory, Peter; and Peel, John. 1977. *Abortion.* Cambridge, England: Cambridge University Press.

Pratt, Gail L.; Koslowsky, Meni; and Wintrob, Ronald M. 1976. Connecticut Physicians' Attitudes toward Abortion. *American Journal of Public Health* 66:288–290.

President's Commission for the Study of Ethical Problems in Medicine and Biomedical and Behavioral Research. 1983. *Screening and Counseling for Genetic Conditions: The Ethical and Social Implications of Genetic Screening, Counseling, and Education Programs.* Washington, D.C.: U.S. Government Printing Office.

Ramsey, Paul. 1978. *Ethics at the Edges of Life: Medical and Legal Intersections.* New Haven: Yale University Press.

Reed, James. 1978. *From Private Vice to Public Virtue: The Birth Control Movement and American Society since 1830.* New York: Basic Books.

Richards, Janet Radcliffe. 1980. *The Skeptical Feminist: A Philosophical Enquiry.* Boston: Routledge & Kegan Paul.

Riesman, David, with Nathan Glazer. 1954. The Meaning of Opinion. In David Riesman, *Individualism Reconsidered and Other Essays*, pp. 492–507. Glencoe, Il.: Free Press.

Robinson, Linda. Abortion Clinic Zoning: The Right to Procreative Freedom and the Zoning Power. 1979. *Women's Rights Law Reporter* 5:283–299.

Rogers, Everett M. [1962]. 1983. *Diffusions of Innovations.* 3d ed. New York: Free Press.

Rongy, Abraham J. 1933. *Abortion: Legal or Illegal?* New York: Vanguard Press.

Rooks, Judith Bourne, and Cates, Jr., Willard. 1977. Emotional Impact of D & E vs. Instillation. *Family Planning Perspectives* 9:276–277.

Rosen, Harold, ed. 1954. *Therapeutic Abortion.* New York: Julian Press.

Rosen, Norma. April 17, 1977. Between Guilt and Gratification. *New York Times Magazine.*

Rosenkrantz, Barbara Gutmann. 1979. Damaged Goods: The Dilemmas of Responsibility for Risk. Millbank Memorial Fund Quarterly/*Health and Society* 57:1–37.

Rosenstock, Irwin M.; Childs, Barton; and Simopoulos, Artemis P. 1975. *Genetic Screening: A Study of the Knowledge and Attitudes of Physicians.* Washington, D.C.: National Academy of Sciences.

Routledge, J. H., Sparling, D. W., and MacFarlane, K. T. 1961. The Present Status of Therapeutic Abortion. *Obstetrics and Gynecology* 17:168–174.

Russell, Keith P. 1951. Therapeutic Abortion in a General Hospital. AJOG 62:434–438.

Sanger, Margaret. *Happiness in Marriage.* [1926]. 1939. New York: Blue Ribbon Books.

Sangmeister, Henry J. 1943. A Survey of Abortion Deaths in Philadelphia from 1931 to 1940 Inclusive. AJOG 46:755–759.

Sarvis, Betty, and Rodman, Hyman. 1974. *The Abortion Controversy.* 2d ed. New York: Columbia University Press.

Scheffel, Carl. 1931. *Medical Jurisprudence.* Philadelphia: P. Blakiston's Son.

Scherman, Quinten. 1958. Therapeutic Abortion. *Obstetrics and Gynecology* 11:323–335.

Schneider, Carl E., and Vinovskis, Maris A., eds. 1980. *The Law and Politics of Abortion.* Lexington, Mass.: D.C. Heath.

Scully, Diana. 1980. *Men Who Control Women's Health: The Miseducation of Obstetrician-Gynecologists.* Boston: Houghton Mifflin.

Seaman, Barbara, and Seaman, Gideon. 1977. *Women and the Crisis in Sex Hormones.* New York: Rawson Associates.

Seims, Sara. 1980. Abortion Availability in the United States. *Family Planning Perspectives* 12:88–101.

Sernett, Milton C. 1980. The Rights of Personhood: The Dred Scott Case and the Question of Abortion. *Religion in Life* 49:461–476.

Shostak, Arthur B., and McLouth, Gary, with Seng, Lynn. 1984. *Men and Abortion: Lessons, Losses, and Love.* New York: Praeger.

Simons, Jalmar H. 1939. Statistical Analysis of One Thousand Abortions. AJOG 37:840–849.

Sloane, R. Bruce, and Horvitz, Diana F. 1974. *A General Guide to Abortion.* Chicago: Nelson-Hall.

State Definitions and Reporting Requirements for Live Births, Fetal Deaths, and Induced Terminations of Pregnancy. [1960, 1966]. 1981. DHHS Publication no. (PHS) 81-1119.

A Statement on Abortion by One Hundred Professors of Obstetrics. 1972. AJOG 112:992–998.

Starr, Paul. 1982. *The Social Transformation of Medicine.* New York: Basic Books.

Steinhoff, Patricia G., and Diamond, Milton. 1977. *Abortion Politics: The Hawaii Experience.* Honolulu: University Press of Hawaii.

Stephenson, Henry A. 1954. Therapeutic Abortion. *Obstetrics and Gynecology* 4:578–580.

Stewart, Phyllis Langton. 1978. A Survey of Obstetrician-Gynecologists' Abortion Attitudes and Performances. *Medical Care* 16:1036–1044.

Stewart, Roger E. 1935. An Analysis of 1,772 Abortions and Miscarriages with a Consideration of Treatment and Prevention. AJOG 29:872–875.

Stone, Martin L.; Gordon, Myron; and Rovinsky, Joseph. 1971. III. The Impact of a Liberalized Abortion Law on the Medical Schools. AJOG 111:728–735.

Strauss, Anselm L., ed. 1973. *Where Medicine Fails.* Rutgers, N.J.: Transaction Books.

Stroh, George, and Hinman, Alan. 1976. Reported Live Births following Induced Abortion: Two and One-half Years' Experience in Upstate New York. AJOG 126:83–90.

Strong, P. M. 1979. *The Ceremonial Order of the Clinic.* London: Routledge & Kegan Paul.

————. 1983. The Rivals: An Essay on the Sociological Trades. In Robert Dingwall and Philip Lewis, eds., *The Sociology of the Professions: Lawyers, Doctors and Others,* pp. 59–77. London: Macmillan.

Stubblefield, Phillip G. 1981. Midtrimester Abortion by Curettage Procedures: An Overview. In Jane E. Hodgson, ed., *Abortion and Sterilization: Medical and Social Aspects.* New York: Grune & Stratton.

Sullivan, Ellen; Tietze, Christopher; and Dryfoos, J. G. 1977. Legal Abortion in the United States, 1975–1976. *Family Planning Perspectives* 9:116–129.

Sun, Marjorie. 1982. Depo-Provera Debate Revs Up at FDA. *Science* 217:424–428.

Taussig, Frederick Joseph. 1910. *The Prevention and Treatment of Abortion.* St. Louis: C. V. Mosby.

————. 1923. *Diseases of the Vulva.* New York: D. Appleton.

————. 1931a. The Abortion Problem in Russia. AJOG 22:134–139.

————. 1931b. Abortion in Relation to Fetal and Maternal Welfare. AJOG 22:868–878.

————. 1934. "Abstract of Discussion" following Clarence O. Cheney, Indications for Therapeutic Abortion: From the Standpoint of the Neurologist and the Psychiatrist. JAMA 103:1918.

————. 1936. *Abortion, Spontaneous and Induced: Medical and Social Aspects.* St. Louis: C. V. Mosby.

————. 1937. Abortion and Its Relation to Fetal and Maternal Mortality. AJOG 33:711–714.

Thomas, Laurence. 1984. Abortion, Slavery, and the Law: A Study in Moral Character. In Jay L. Garfield and Patricia Hennessey, eds., *Abortion: Moral and Legal Perspectives,* pp. 227–237. Amherst, Mass.: University of Massachusetts Press.

Thomson, Judith Jarvis. [1971]. 1974. A Defense of Abortion. In Marshall Cohen, Thomas Nagel, and Thomas Scanlon, eds., *The Rights and Wrongs of Abortion,* pp. 3–22. Princeton: Princeton University Press.

Thornton, Jr., W. N. 1953. Therapeutic Abortion: Responsibility of the Obstetrician. *Obstetrics and Gynecology* 2:470–475.

Tietze, Christopher. 1948. An Investigation into the Incidence of Abortion in Baltimore. AJOG 56:1160–1162.

———. 1950. Therapeutic Abortions in New York City, 1943–1947. AJOG 60:146–152.

———. 1976. Incidence of Legal Abortion. In Abdel R. Omran, ed., *Liberalization of Abortion Laws: Implications*, pp. 1–17. Chapel Hill, N.C.: Carolina Population Center, University of North Carolina at Chapel Hill.

Tooley, Michael. 1983. *Abortion and Infanticide*. Oxford: Clarendon Press.

Tschetter, Paul. 1978. Family Planning and the Primary Care Physician. *Family Planning Perspectives* 10:350–353.

Tyler, Jr., Carl W. 1981. Epidemiology of Abortion. *Journal of Reproductive Medicine* 26:459–469.

Vetterling-Braggin, Mary; Elliston, Frederick A.; and English, Jane, eds. 1977. *Feminism and Philosophy*. Totowa, N.J.: Littlefield, Adams.

Wagner, Sonia. 1978. Woman's Right, Physician's Judgment: *Commonwealth v. Edelin* and a Physician's Criminal Liability for Fetal Manslaughter. *Women's Rights Law Reporter* 4:97–114.

Walbert, David F., and Butler, J. Douglas, eds. 1973. *Abortion, Society, and the Law*. Cleveland: The Press of Case Western Reserve University.

Walters, William, and Singer, Peter, eds. 1982. *Test-Tube Babies: A Guide to Moral Questions, Present Techniques and Future Possibilities*. New York: Oxford University Press.

Wardle, Lynn D. 1980. *The Abortion Privacy Doctrine: A Compendium and Critique of Federal Court Abortion Cases*. Buffalo: William S. Hein.

Watkins, Raymond E. 1933. A Five-Year Study of Abortion. AJOG 25:161–172.

Wattleton, Faye, and Kissling, Frances. March 11, 1978. Letter to the Editor. This Is the Central Story of Legal Abortion. *New York Times*, p. 22.

Weber, Max. [1919]. 1948. Science as a Vocation. In H. H. Gerth and C. Wright Mills, eds., *From Max Weber: Essays in Sociology*, pp. 129–156. London: Routledge & Kegan Paul.

Wechsler, Henry. 1976. *Handbook of Medical Specialties*. New York: Human Sciences Press.

Weisman, Abner I. 1972. Open Legal Abortion "On Request" Is Working in New York City, But Is It the Answer? AJOG 112:138–143.

Wertheimer, Roger. 1977. Philosophy on Humanity. In Edward Manier, William Liu, and David Solomon, eds., *Abortion: New Directions for Policy Studies*, pp. 117–136. Notre Dame, Ind.: University of Notre Dame Press.

Wile, Ira S., ed. 1934. *The Sex Life of the Unmarried Adult: An Inquiry into and an Interpretation of Current Sex Practices*. New York: Vanguard Press.

Wolf, Sanford R.; Sasaki, Tom T.; and Cushner, Irvin M. 1971. Assumption of Attitudes toward Abortion during Physician Education. *Obstetrics and Gynecology* 37:141–147.

Wolff, John R.; Nielson, Paul E.; and Schiller, Patricia J. 1971. Therapeutic Abortion: Attitudes of Medical Personnel Leading to Complications in Patient Care. AJOG 110:730–733.

Dr. X as Told to Lucy Freeman. 1962. *The Abortionist*. Garden City, N.Y.: Doubleday.

Zatuchni, G. I.; Sciarra, J. J.; and Speidel, J. J., eds. 1979. *Pregnancy Termination: Procedures, Safety, and New Developments*. Hagerstown, Md.: Harper & Row.

Zerubavel, Eviatar. 1981. *Hidden Rhythms: Schedules and Calendars in Social Life*. Chicago: University of Chicago Press.

Zimmerman, Mary K. 1977. *Passage through Abortion: The Personal and Social Reality of Women's Experiences*. New York: Praeger.

Index

Abortion: access to, xii, 14, 23–24, 31, 65; and religion, 2, 12, 15, 17, 43–46, 71; criminal and illegal, 4, 7–8, 9, 12, 22, 119; as a form of birth control, 4, 7, 32–33, 35, 122, 146n2; legalization of, 7, 29, 77, 118; and hospital policy, 15, 44; as a right, 20, 23, 123; and the poor, 27, 31; and social policy, 35, 121, 123; in-office, 48, 54, 59; risks associated with, 64, 117, 120, 122; routinization of, 78, 79, 90, 121, 124

Abortion, elective. *See* Elective abortion

Abortion, first-trimester. *See* First-trimester abortion(s)

Abortion, indications for. *See* Indications for abortion

Abortion, second-trimester. *See* Second-trimester abortion(s)

Abortion, therapeutic. *See* Therapeutic abortion

Abortion clinics. *See* Clinic(s)

Abortionist, 2, 14, 62, 70, 120; stigma of, 68–69, 84

Abortion kits, 66, 117

Abortion referral. *See* Referral(s)

Adair, F. L., 12

Adams, Dr. (pseudonym), 62–63, 66–67

American Board of Obstetrics and Gynecology, 41–42

American College of Obstetricians and Gynecologists, 30, 66

American Medical Association, 2, 10, 22

Amniocentesis, 65, 104–106, 108, 111, 145n6

Bates, Jerome E., 4

Beal v. Doe, 66, 142n7

Becker, Howard S., 110

Becker, Marshall H., 118

Behrman, Richard E., 88

Bioethics, ix, 34–36, 104

Birth control, 1, 11, 47–48, 65, 115; right to, 21, 120; politics of, 27, 37, 50, 52; counseling, 43, 46, 49, 50–51, 54; benefits and risks, 107

Birth control movement, 1, 6–7, 10, 11, 32, 120

Birth control services, 37, 43, 70

Blake, Judith, 30

Board certification, 41–43, 93, 112

Bosk, Charles, 76

Boynton, M. W., 12

Calling, 55, 74; of physician, 11, 101–102, 111; to medicine, 94, 97, 98, 101, 110. *See also* Vocation

Caplow, Theodore, 114

Carter, Patricia A., 15–18 passim

Central Hospital (pseudonym), 38

Choice (referral service), 40

Clinic(s): culture of, x, xii, 34, 73, 93, 117, 122; vs. private practice, 9, 32, 37, 76, 112; abortion, 30, 62, 114,

161